DATE DUE

DEC 1 8 1998	
GAYLORD	PRINTED IN U.S.A.

PRESCRIPTION FOR PROFIT

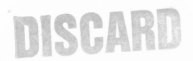

PRESCRIPTION FOR PROFIT

How Doctors Defraud Medicaid

PAUL JESILOW, HENRY N. PONTELL,
AND GILBERT GEIS

UNIVERSITY OF CALIFORNIA PRESS
BERKELEY   LOS ANGELES   LONDON

The research presented here was funded by grants from the University of California, Irvine; Indiana University; and the National Institute of Justice, U.S. Department of Justice (#82-1J-CX-0035).

University of California Press
Berkeley and Los Angeles, California

University of California Press, Ltd.
London, England

Library of Congress Cataloging-in-Publication Data
Jesilow, Paul, 1950–
    Prescription for profit : how doctors defraud Medicaid / Paul
Jesilow, Henry N. Pontell, and Gilbert Geis.
        p.   cm.
    Includes bibliographical references.
    ISBN 0-520-07614-1 (cloth : alk. paper)
    1. Medicaid fraud.   2. Physicians—Malpractice—United States.
I. Pontell, Henry N., 1950–   .   II. Geis, Gilbert.   III. Title.
    [DNLM: 1. Fraud.   2. Insurance Claim Reporting—United States.
3. Medicaid.   4. Physicians.   W 275 AA1 J5p]
RA412.5.U6J47   1993
364.1'63—dc20
DNLM/DLC
for Library of Congress   91-36944
                                                                 CIP

Printed in the United States of America
1   2   3   4   5   6   7   8   9

The paper used in this publication meets the minimum requirements of American National Standard for Information Sciences—Permanence of Paper for Printed Library Materials, ANSI Z39.48-1984. ⊚

For our families

Contents

Preface

The world of medicine has been of compelling personal and professional interest to the three authors of this book for some time. Paul Jesilow underwent lengthy hospital stays because of a spinal cord injury at the time when the government medical benefit programs—Medicaid and Medicare—were beginning to bring about basic changes in how physicians practiced their profession. In graduate school in the 1970s, Henry Pontell worked at a large medical school as the research director on a project concerned with the delivery of emergency medical care. Gilbert Geis has a collection of news reports dating from the 1950s on matters such as fee-splitting among doctors and the involvement of fringe practitioners in illegal abortions.

The three of us also have had close contact with many medical doctors, both as their patients and as their friends. The University of California, Irvine, has a medical school, and we have worked in various capacities with some of its faculty and developed great respect for their dedication and skill. We have collectively logged more than enough time in the role of patients and share a deep sense of gratitude to individual physicians. For Jesilow, his family physician, Daniel B. Beck, M.D., represents the kind of doctor made immortal in American folklore: wise, caring, and much more concerned with the welfare of his patients than the well-being of his purse. Steve Reynard, M.D., Geis's doctor, when told about the nature of this study, immediately responded, "Nail those bastards." His own dedication to the best traditions of medicine—the time he spends and the concern he shows—

seems awesome to a sociologist who has watched him at work for several decades now. The late Tibor Nyilas, M.D., Pontell's family physician for over twenty years, is fondly remembered as a doctor of the highest compassion, honesty, and skill.

We also have had personal experiences with the downside of medical practice. That experience was inevitably heightened as we carried out our study of Medicaid fraud. We have tried throughout this book to avoid heavy-handed depictions of all doctors with the brush that paints in dark colors the depredations of some. That task is considerably more difficult than it might appear. If one studies burglars, citizens who avoid breaking into others' homes do not feel that *their* reputations are being endangered. But if one reports on frauds committed by doctors, the vast majority of doctors, whose conduct is honest and aboveboard, none-theless are tempted to complain that their entire profession is being unfairly besmirched. So we underscore here that our topic is limited to doctors who cheat, and our case studies and interviews focus on doctors who have been found guilty or have pled guilty to cheating Medicaid and been punished for their offenses. Besides creating an inventory of medical frauds, we seek to understand something about the doctors who perpetrate them: who they are, what they do, how they are caught, and how they respond to what happens to them. In the course of this portrayal, we hope to explain what is taking place—that is, why doctors, who in the past rarely came into contact with criminal law because of irregular professional practices, now are much more often in that position.

The first two chapters establish a context for understanding the case studies and interview material. Among other matters, we discuss various earlier (and at times continuing) forms of crime by medical doctors, the considerable tension between the practice of medicine as a profession and as a business, and the significant changes wrought in both of those aspects of medical work by the appearance of Medicare and Medicaid. We also examine the sad discordance between the original ideals en-visioned for Medicaid and the bleak consequences of later concerns about dramatically escalating costs.

In chapter 3 we present the results of our interviews with federal, state, and private officials regarding the enforcement problems with which they have had to cope. Chapter 4 details, from case file information, the kinds of offenses that result in formal investigations and criminal charges. In chapter 5 we quote extensively from our interviews with apprehended violators to demonstrate how these doctors regard what happened to them and how they see the Medicaid program. In our concluding chapter we attempt to clarify some of the causes of physician fraud by comparing Medicare and Medicaid to the national health care programs in Britain, Canada, and Australia. We also speculate about the possible significance of recent trends in American health care, including the corporatization of medicine and the rising number of women entering medicine.

We owe a great deal of thanks to the scores of persons who have helped us during the nearly ten years in which we have been at work on this project. Foremost among these are Mary Jane O'Brien, our executive assistant during the period we received funding from the National Institute of Justice of the United States Department of Justice, the University of California, Irvine, and Indiana University. Steve Rosoff and Connie Keenan were exemplary graduate research assistants who helped us in many tasks, including our interviews with doctors.

Many students provided us with seemingly endless data and literature from library searches. We thank all of them for their hard work and support, especially Stan Pennington, "Stash" Baronett, John Espar, Audrey Shelton, Damian A. Moreno, William Grenner, Sally Sun, Cindy Jenner, Anna Pisani, Pam Shelly, and Peggy Cherry.

We also thank the individuals at various federal and state agencies and the many physicians who consented to be interviewed and provided us with insights about Medicaid fraud by doctors. To ensure the anonymity we promised them, they and their organizations must remain nameless.

Finally, we thank the staff at the University of California, Irvine, and the staff at Indiana University for their tireless work. This book would not have been completed without the help of Carol Wyatt, Judy Omiya, Mirella Marinelli, Katherine O'Neil, Judy Kelly, and Claudia Lavenant.

Chapter One

Professional Entrepreneurs

The inauguration of federally financed Medicare and Medicaid programs created new opportunities for fraud and abuse by members of the medical profession. Physicians had been beguiled into accepting the federal benefit programs—though as a group they kicked and screamed along the way—because they presumed they could control the direction the programs would take. The benefit programs had come about in response to restiveness among voters, particularly among the growing ranks of the elderly, who feared that they would be impoverished by overwhelming medical expenses. For the medical profession, it seemed wiser to assuage such fears with concessions rather than risk more serious threats to its autonomy should the public demand even stronger relief.

It should have been obvious from the beginning that the president and the Congress, responsible for funding the medical benefit programs, would sooner or later demand fiscal accountability. It should also have been obvious that doctors would lose professional autonomy as the way they practiced and set their fees came under the scrutiny of nonmedical overseers. For these watchdogs, quality of care is not the overriding priority. They have to balance demands on government resources while placating competing constituencies and, in particular, striving to maintain their own incumbencies.

In this book we identify crucial issues in the attitudes and structure of the medical profession as they relate to the enforcement of laws and regulations concerned with fraud and abuse in Medicaid, a predominantly state-funded program administered largely for the benefit of the needy. (Medicare, in contrast, is federally funded and designed for the elderly.) The inauguration of these programs created new kinds of medical malefactors. There would be no gain, for instance, in performing extensive diagnostic tests on a poor person unable to pay for them; but if an insurer will meet the charges, there is a great deal to be garnered by doing such work, needed or not, and by doing it as cheaply as possible. No one has been able to calculate the precise cost of fraud and abuse associated with Medicare and Medicaid, but every year about two hundred physicians are suspended from participation in these programs because of fraudulent or abusive practices. Such practices include submitting bills for X rays done without film, blood and urine specimens that were never analyzed, and treatments much different—and more expensive—from those actually carried out.

Physicians punished for Medicaid violations typically do not represent the mainstream of U.S. medicine. They are marginal within the profession, not necessarily because of their abilities but because of characteristics of their practices or of themselves. About one-third graduated from foreign medical schools; blacks and psychiatrists are also overrepresented. The demographic portrait of physicians sanctioned by Medicaid is strongly affected by enforcement strategies, which tend to focus on doctors practicing in poor neighborhoods. We discuss the bases for this situation more fully in chapter 4.

THE ADVENT OF
HEALTH INSURANCE

The American Medical Association (AMA) campaigned mightily in the early 1960s against government benefit programs; today the association is fighting limitations that might be imposed on the programs. A newspaper reporter notes, for instance, that years ago the actor Ronald Reagan made a recording to help the AMA "with its greatest fight: the no-holds-barred effort to halt the 'socialist threat of Medicare.'" As president, Reagan was "still in the thick of that fray, trying to curb spending on the federal health programs that he and the doctors' lobby were unable to block." But Reagan's former allies now had changed

sides. "Enough is enough," the AMA declared in full-page advertisements, urging Congress not to cut the budgets of the health programs.
"At heart the AMA hasn't really changed at all. It is still pursuing its
139-year-old mission to preserve the *freedom* and *income* of doctors."[1]

The recollections of Jimmy Carter also illustrate how a shift in
position can alter a person's attitude toward medical spending. Carter
had served on the Sumter County Hospital Authority in Georgia before
he went into electoral politics. At the beginning of his term as president,
he regretted the local policies he had once supported:

I have seen in retrospect, from a little different perspective, that we were
naturally inclined to buy a new machine whenever it became available and
then to mandate, to require that every patient who came into the hospital had
to submit to a blood sample or some other aspect of their body to the machine
for analysis, whether they needed it or not, in order to rapidly defray the cost
of the purchase of the machine. I did not realize that I was ripping off people,
never thought about it too much. It was a fact.[2]

With practitioners' ability to control their own operations greatly
reduced under Medicaid, some physicians have pushed against the new
restraints in unauthorized, illegal ways. Behaviors that would have gone
unnoted in earlier years now lead to difficulties with the law. In addition, large numbers of new physician scams have come into being.

Before the advent of Medicaid, doctors routinely discriminated
among patients with regard to fees. In metropolitan areas, where physicians often did not know their clients personally, people commonly
wore shabby clothing and left jewelry and other indications of financial
well-being behind when visiting doctors' offices. Doctors typically justified their soaking of the rich as a reasonable method to permit them
to treat the poor who could not afford the customary fees. These tactics
fell in line with the Hippocratic oath, the ethical demand on medical
practitioners that they selflessly make their professional skills available
to all those in need.

This crude sort of economic justice was practicable because there was
no sense that any given medical activity was worth a stipulated and
settled sum and that the sum ought to be the same for all patients.
Occasionally a doctor would be chastised for an excessive fee, as when

William Halsted—a founder of Johns Hopkins University—charged $10,000 for a surgery.[3] But overall, an important element of decency underlay the tactic of variable fees: Doctors were not exploiting patients indifferently; they were, with some semblance of fairness, merely determining who could afford to pay a premium for their services. Undoubtedly, those persons who paid higher fees often received better service. They were the kinds of patients worth satisfying, and they probably also demanded more.

Doctors' autonomy permitted them to proceed unchallenged by all but raw marketplace considerations in the pursuit of their financial self-interest. That doctors could determine to some extent what they earned did not arouse much soul-searching. For one thing, competition among healers helped establish a "reasonable" income for doctors. For another, the sums doctors were making were not usually regarded as unconscionable—in part because the services they offered fell far short of the dazzling and marvelously successful panoply of treatments available today.

Ironically, as doctors' ability to keep people alive and healthy reaches impressive new heights, the profession is losing prestige. Before the turn of the century, most doctors in the United States did not enjoy a particularly high social standing. Medical treatment had little to offer the sick. Opiates helped alleviate suffering, but other heroic procedures—such as bloodletting, oral doses of mercury, and septic surgeries—often worsened rather than improved the patient's condition. As one historian points out, "until well into the twentieth century, really until the end of the 1930s, formal medicine was largely impotent in the face of serious disease. The doctor could reassure the patient and console the relatives, but he was biologically as ineffective, if socially as necessary, as the parson or undertaker."[4]

Before the 1920s the sick often did not go to physicians for medical attention. Home remedies, best known to the neighborhood women, were routinely administered. The hospital was a place where poor people went to die and where some physicians learned their relatively few skills by practicing on these paupers. The hospitals were run as charity institutions in response to a religious sense of moral obligation.[5]

The role and standing of the physician and the hospital began to change noticeably at the turn of the last century. Lister's emphasis on aseptic surgery and Pasteur's and Koch's work on bacteria offered the hope that medicine might cure disease and other ailments. As a result, the value of medical services increased. The rising cost of medical achievements during the first three decades of the twentieth century necessitated a financial alliance between doctors and hospitals.[6] Hospitals purchased equipment that was too costly for the individual practitioner. The best-equipped health care facilities could then lure the finest physicians, who in turn attracted the wealthiest patients.

By the period of the Depression, from 1929 onward, persons from all social classes began to patronize hospitals in larger numbers, paying, on sliding scales, their "fair" share of the cost of the facility and the physicians' fees. Patient care also tended to be on a sliding scale, degenerating in some instances to neglect of those who could not purchase better treatment. In 1932 a report funded by eight philanthropic foundations documented the disparity in medical and hospital care in terms of the wealth of the patient; costs were also keeping working-class people from seeking medical attention when they required it.[7] The poor increasingly began to be shunted off to county and university hospitals to be used as mannequins for the education of aspiring physicians.

The Great Depression galvanized changes in how Americans paid for their health care and in the financial arrangements of medical practice. The new diagnostic and treatment facilities in the hospitals required additional funds and stable income sources; yet receipts from patients were declining. Voluntary health insurance, such as Blue Cross, emerged as the mechanism to allow patients to meet escalating hospital bills, but the cost of ever-newer technology and of maintaining expensive equipment continued to drive up hospital fees.[8]

Indeed, hospitals could spend freely with the assurance that Blue Cross would reimburse them because physicians and hospitals controlled the insurance programs. By 1938 the American Hospital Association (AHA) and the Blue Cross Association (BCA) had established an interlocking directorate. The BCA selected two members of the AHA Board of Directors, and the AHA designated three members for the BCA board.[9] The AHA controlled the standards for the approval of Blue

Cross plans, and the rules it promulgated essentially placed control of the Blue Cross program in the hands of hospital physicians.[10]

The Blue Shield plans, which provided third-party insurance for physician services, began to grow during the 1940s. The AMA exercised strict control over this and other prepayment plans because physicians feared the insurance schemes might jeopardize their elite status, threaten incomes, and invade professional autonomy. Particularly worrisome was the thought that prepayment plans would introduce uniform pricing for medical services. To forestall that possibility, the AMA made a number of demands: For a Blue Shield plan to be accepted by the AMA, doctors had to control all aspects of medical services, including diagnosis, treatment, and costs. The AMA also barred any insurer from intruding between patients and physicians. Patients were to be free to select any participating physician, and their medical relationships with these physicians were to remain confidential. Finally, the AMA required that patients' premiums be tied to their incomes.[11] (As we will see, the AMA insisted on many of the same concessions in the debates over Medicaid and Medicare.)

The AMA-dictated blueprint for Blue Shield thus enabled hospitals and physicians to establish their own prices and to assure that their bills would be paid. Layperson involvement in the process of medical care and pricing was effectively hamstrung.

Early on, both Blue Cross and Blue Shield had problems with overutilization of services by patients as well as fraud and abuse by physicians.[12] Adding deductibles seemed to curb the first problem, but the second remained largely unaddressed, in part because costs could be passed along to customers each year in the form of premium hikes.

The advent of Medicare and Medicaid, however, dramatically altered conditions for doctors. Changes in how they are paid have caused many American doctors to come to believe that their profession has lost the social and economic status that made it so attractive in the past. Doctors believe that their authority and independence have been eroded by government officials, insurers, corporate managers, and hospital administrators. As an orthopedic surgeon noted, "It's not so much fun to practice medicine as it was twenty years ago. The judgment of physicians has been usurped by cookbook criteria created by people who are not doctors." The proportion of U.S. doctors who are salaried employees at hospitals, clinics, and other health care organizations is rising each year (from 23.4 percent in 1983 to 27 percent in 1988, for example). Among physicians under the age of thirty-six, 47 percent are employees, compared to 19 percent of those fifty-five years and older. In Minneapolis, doctors threatened to unionize, a move said to be dictated "by rising frustration over the dramatic changes sweeping the health care industry that are eroding their authority and income."[13]

Doctors' earnings put them in the top 3 percent of the American working population. In 1987 physicians' median incomes increased 6.5 percent, far outstripping inflation, to almost $120,000 annually after expenses but before taxes. The AMA claimed the rise was due to longer hours and the performance of more surgical procedures. But consumer advocates called the income increase "scandalous" and claimed that doctors' overcharges of programs such as Medicare were "outrageous." A public opinion poll in 1984 found that only 27 percent of the public felt that doctors' fees were "usually reasonable," compared to 42 percent who had felt that way two years earlier. Sarcasm, generally spared medical practitioners, was coming into play: "It's not like they're living on the brink of poverty" was the response to the income figures by Dr. Sidney Wolfe, director of the Public Citizen Health Group.[14]

The interplay between how medicine is practiced and profit incentives was highlighted by a Congressional Budget Office report suggesting that "physicians may sometimes respond to economic pressures" by attempting to "induce patients to consume additional medical services, whose expected benefits would be small." When patients cut down on the number of their visits, one study demonstrated, some physicians responded by encouraging them to use more services. Outside analysts thought such tactics ultimately would be self-defeating. A professor of political economy at Princeton University suggested that physicians could play "that game" for a few more years, but soon the less costly services of nurse-practitioners and other paramedics would displace those of medical doctors.[15]

The fee-for-service reimbursement approach of government medical benefit programs provides the basis for doctors to increase income illegally with little risk of apprehension. Because doctors are reimbursed a fixed amount for each procedure, they can earn additional income by charging for a more expensive procedure than the one performed, double-billing for services, pingponging (sending patients back and forth for unnecessary visits), family ganging (examining all members of the family in one visit), churning (mandating unnecessary visits), and prolonging treatments.

The fee-for-service reimbursement has been pinpointed as a major contributor to the disintegration of standards among physicians:

Fee-for-service medicine subtly corrupts its own practitioners. Motives for entering medicine are many and complex but the strongest is the desire to be a healer. . . . Unfortunately, the feelings of dominance that inevitably accompany the healer's role frequently overpower whatever native idealism a doctor might have brought to his profession. The grueling 100-hour weeks spent as a resident encourage him to feel unappreciated for his important work. As he gets older, he also begins believing that the same power and respect he commands in the office or operating room should extend into the community, where the badges of success and status, instead of centering on the value of one's work, center on material possessions and social standing. And as the fee-for-service system combines with the doctor's revered status to make these things accessible, what increasingly becomes important are not the satisfactions of medicine but the benefits that result from practicing it. For these doctors, stories of million-dollar incomes do not provoke outrage, but envy.[16]

In their battle to retain fee-for-service reimbursement, doctors often insist that inroads on their autonomy erode the quality of patient care. But this view, accurate or not, carries less and less weight in the battle with brute economic forces. Patients with the wherewithal remain able to buy the best care on the market, while politicians are increasingly unmoved by a plea that carries so heavy a load of physician self-interest.

Complaints about a deterioration in medical services because of government-dictated rules clearly are not altogether without merit. The payment schedules used by the government-financed programs, for example, place a premium on performing certain tasks and not others. But those nonpaid services can be equally or more important for the patient's welfare. As Norman Cousins has pointed out, the work of a physician now comes under "computer appraisal" and there is no dollar return "for the time spent in taking a detailed history and doing a slow and purposeful physical examination, and above all making the patient understand what has been done, why it has been done, and what is the appropriate health care program."[17]

Dr. Stuart S. Howards, a urology professor at the University of Virginia, sees a particular change in the way physicians regard what he believes was at one time more a calling than a trade: "Physicians are being reduced to businessmen." A retired physician puts the matter another way: "Once, being a doctor was a noble profession. But in the last years, it became a job."

Doctoring, of course, has always possessed business and professional elements in uneasy alignment. Three hundred years ago Sir Samuel Garth also thought that a proud profession was being transformed into a sordid commercial enterprise: "Now sickening Physick [medicine] hangs her pensive head. And what was once a Science, now's a trade."[18] The accelerating pace of physician embourgeoisement (although on a grand bourgeois scale), however, is provoking considerable dissatisfaction among practitioners today.

This dual nature of the practice of medicine—its joint business and professional character—makes it something of a schizophrenic, or at least an ambiguous, enterprise. It is, of course, not unique in this regard; most notably, the private practice of law shares essentially the same characteristic. Lawyering, of course, has come to be defined fiscally in the public mind as an aggressively self-interested pursuit; and the now-constant battles between doctors and lawyers in malpractice liability suits likely has tarnished the image of both groups. That lawyers still peer jealously at the position of doctors is reflected in the title of a recent article in the *American Bar Association Journal*: "MD Salaries Rise Again—Easily Surpassing Lawyers."[19]

Money made by the practice of law, however, unlike that realized in medicine, is primarily derived directly from clients; the services provided by a lawyer, therefore, are justified on the basis of a financial (rather than a health) cost-benefit equation: the client has to gain more money, or be safeguarded against the loss of more money, than the attorney demands as a fee.

The autonomy of attorneys is also considerably checked by the fact that the most remunerative work goes to large firms, which are structured in hierarchical form and demand what often is a trying period of apprenticeship without a sure guarantee of a partnership. Lawyers also are subservient to judicial control.

Nonetheless, the theme of economic purity heard in regard to medicine also appears regularly in legal discussions. A former president of the American Bar Association, for instance, has called for a rededication to "principle" over "profit" and to "professionalism" over "commercialism."[20] The most distinctive structural difference in regard to crimes committed in the course of their work by lawyers and by physicians is that lawyers are not controlled by federal and state funding agencies. Lawyers still rely on policing themselves, as doctors once did. All states but Alabama and Maine, for instance, have funds, primarily derived from dues charged to practicing lawyers, that compensate victims of attorneys' misdeeds. A newspaper story illustrates how such a system can cover up what may be endemic cheating and define the derelictions in "bad apple" terms, a tactic often used by the medical profession as well: "Most of these deviant lawyers are graduates of marginal law schools, eking out livings from vulnerable clients. Many of them are alcoholics, gamblers, or cocaine addicts. Invariably they cannot make restitution themselves because they have been disbarred or imprisoned, are broke, or have disappeared."[21]

Lawyers also tend to work in public or semipublic arenas, where their actions may be more scrupulously examined. But, basically, it is the monitoring of doctors and lawyers, as well as the different kinds of laws and rules applied to them, that makes the record of their criminal behavior different. Besides, the practice of medicine has enjoyed a much more exalted status than that of law. Only recently has the taint of money—"filthy lucre," as the medieval church fathers denominated that ungodly commodity—become unpleasantly associated with doctors. At the same time, the income of physicians contributes to their status. Astronomic earnings both appall and appeal to the average citizen.

Numerous studies document the high standing of physicians in America through the years. In 1925 one researcher presented a list of forty-five occupations to high school seniors, college freshmen, and schoolteachers and asked them to rank the occupations in order of their prestige. Physicians were ranked third highest, behind bankers and ministers. Ten years later, in an ordering of forty-one occupations by high school students, physicians were second, behind clergymen. Physicians were at the head of the list in six subsequent studies.[22] In the 1940s the National Opinion Research Center presented a list of ninety occupations to a representative national sample of 2,900 persons. Physicians finished in a tie for second place with state governors, surpassed only by U.S. Supreme Court justices. More recently, a Gallup poll found doctors outpacing the clergy, college professors, and business executives (in that order) among occupations designated "very prestigious."[23]

High status can insulate its holders from public condemnation—to a point. But once that threshold is passed, the public can be especially condemnatory of fallen idols. People may feel they have been sold out or tricked and thus may react more strongly. Such a process of public response will be of particular concern when we examine frauds by physicians against medical benefit programs.

Typically, doctors are politically conservative. They strongly believe in individual effort unfettered by governmental constraints, and many of them will point to their own success as testimony to the virtue of their political principles. This ideological opposition to government interference prompts some doctors to cheat medical aid programs with impunity and later protest that they have been bedeviled and viciously persecuted by unholy forces. Convicted physicians often insist that their crimes were merely the consequence of their being too involved in heady medical matters to attend to the niggling red tape of the programs that were paying them. This not uncommon strain of professional arrogance among medical practitioners may help the guilty deflect the disgrace of criminal prosecutions, the accompanying unpleasant publicity, and assaults on their self-esteem.[24] The same arrogance may also contribute to behaviors that lead to wrongdoing in the first place.

Sir William Osler, the preeminent medical figure of the nineteenth century, attributed such arrogance to the fact that doctors' work often lacks leavening influences: "No class of men needs friction so much as physicians—no class gets less. The daily round of a busy practitioner tends to develop an egotism of a most intense kind, to which there is no antidote. The few setbacks are forgotten, the mistakes are often buried, and ten years of successful work tends to make a man touchy, dogmatic, intolerant of correction, and abominably self-centered." According to his biographer, Osler, commenting on the conflict between service and self-serving behavior, "even seemed to go so far as to think that a man could not make more than a bare living and still be an honest and competent physician."[25]

At the same time, doctors offer services that can be regarded as literally priceless: Without what they do, more people would die more quickly, and in the light of this consideration other concerns pale into insignificance. "Your money or your life," a thief commanded Jack Benny in one of his skits. The audience laughed when Benny, assuming his public persona as a tightwad, hesitated, apparently unable to decide which option was preferable. "I'm thinking, I'm thinking," Benny said, a tone of nervous uncertainty in his voice. But we know immediately what our choice would be—no amount of money is worth death. Therein lies a great source of physicians' power and an important correlate of crimes by doctors in the course of their work.

These, then, are the matters with which we will be concerned in this book. We seek to document forms and degrees of the "new crimes" by doctors, focusing in particular on crimes committed against the Medicaid program, which was instituted in 1965 primarily as a heroic attempt to bring mainstream medical care to those unable to afford it.

The extent of crimes perpetrated by physicians against Medicaid is unknown. Estimates range from 10 percent to 25 percent of the total program cost[26]—which in 1989 was $61 billion—but we have not found any evidence to support either figure. On this topic, little has changed since 1977, when the director of the Congressional Budget Office (CBO) was asked to comment on the financial implications of a bill creating investigative units to concentrate on fraud against the benefit programs. She replied, "The unknown magnitude of fraud and abuse presently extant in the programs makes it impracticable for the CBO to project the actual cost impact of this measure at this time."[27]

Certainly, some of the violations have been extraordinary, even bizarre. In Illinois, a psychiatrist billed Medicaid for forty-eight hundred hours in the year, or almost twenty-four hours each workday.[28] Other doctors have been caught billing for services on persons who were dead at the time the alleged work was performed. An optometrist sold patients cataract lenses for $35 and charged the government $180 for reading glasses. A doctor billed Medicaid for $3,000 for office procedures on dates when he was in Africa on a safari. An ophthalmologist performed unnecessary eye operations that left fourteen persons with impaired vision in a scheme that defrauded the state of $14,000. A psychiatrist charged Medicaid for sexual liaisons with a patient, claiming he had submitted the bills for professional services so his wife, who handled his books, would not become suspicious.

Another doctor billed for abortions on women who were not pregnant, including one who had had a hysterectomy. In forty-eight separate instances, he billed Medicaid for performing two abortions within a month on the same patient. In a most unusual case during the early days of the program, a Florida physician, identified as the top biller in the state, was found to have requested payment for treating a twenty-two-year-old college football player for diaper rash. Ultimately, the doctor received a twenty-year sentence for fraud. A life sentence was added when she was convicted of hiring someone to kill her partner to prevent him from testifying in the Medicaid case.[29]

Other health care providers have been no less bizarre than physicians in their Medicaid billing habits. Ambulance services have billed for round-trip transportation for patients who died en route to the hospital. A dentist billed for extracting thirty-eight teeth from a single patient (the average adult mouth contains only thirty-two teeth).[30]

CRIME AND PROFESSIONAL ENTREPRENEURSHIP

It is an axiom of capitalism that financial self-interest will compel people to perform in ways that ultimately benefit us all. The spirit of capitalism also often leads people to equate who they are—their self-esteem—with how much they earn. Almost a century ago, Emile Durkheim, the preeminent French sociologist, observed that the unchecked spiral of ambition can account for illegal acquisitive behavior by those who seemingly have little need for further accumulation: "Overweaning ambition always exceeds the results obtained. Striving for the unattainable is for them pleasure in itself."[31] But the drive to acquire also prevails in noncapitalist societies. In Communist Poland, for instance, patients had to bribe doctors if they desired to be treated expeditiously.[32] Whether some degree of greed is an inherent feature of human nature or an acquired characteristic is arguable; that it exists throughout the industrialized world is evident. What we have and what we want influence how we act, as do opportunity, conscience, and the dictates of our upbringing and experiences. The likelihood of being caught at wrongdoing and the consequences also bear on how we behave.

For American doctors, what has increased dramatically in recent years are the opportunities for painless financial self-aggrandizement and, concomitantly, the strength of the barriers (the law enforcement presence) dedicated to controlling such self-aggrandizement.

In describing the social structure of the doctor-patient relationship, Talcott Parsons, in a classic analysis, noted the importance that the medical profession places on the ideal of "selflessness" in dealing with patients. The ideology of the medical profession emphasizes the physician's obligation to put the patient's welfare above the doctor's personal interests. "Commercialism" is regarded as the most serious and insidious evil with which the profession has to contend.[33] The "profit motive" is supposed to be excluded from the world of medicine. This attitude is, of course, shared with the other professions, but Parsons found it more pronounced in the medical realm than anywhere else, except perhaps among the clergy. Selfless professionalism, Parsons noted, including affective neutrality, helps define the doctor's role in society. But even as it enables doctors to enter into patients' private lives, it also provides a protective cloak from outside scrutiny.

Traditionally, any deviations in medical practice were handled through informal channels rather than by formal control mechanisms. With informal channels, Parsons stated, physicians could gain more confidence and use more "daring" interventions in attempts to help patients than might be allowed in a bureaucratically controlled situation, where review of "technical aspects" might stifle innovation. Although a certain amount of abuse got by, both altruistic and self-interested elements of motivation provided social control within the profession. In Parsons's view, "it is to a physician's self-interest to act contrary to his own self-interest—in an immediate situation, of course, not in the long run."[34] By embracing the ideology of "selflessness" in immediate situations, physicians could ensure their long-term self-interests of professional hegemony, high financial rewards, and relative autonomy.

Parsons's portrait of the structure and function of the practice of medicine in the United States combines a shrewd appraisal of key elements with a conservative bias that accepts too uncritically the position that extant conditions persist because they are functional and in the best interests of the social system. He probably was correct, though, in perceiving that as long as medicine remained beyond the oversight of other self-interested and powerful agencies, its reputation would stay untainted, and its procedures could simultaneously serve practitioners' interests and those of most patients as well.

Until the advent of Medicare and Medicaid, medical practitioners had to decide, without significant external scrutiny, between their professional obligations and their financial interests. A particularly pointed example of the tensions between the demands of a professional calling and the dictates of financial self-interest is the situation of pharmacists.[35] A study by Richard Quinney of the value orientations of twenty pharmacists who had been caught for prescription violations and sixty pharmacists with clean records found a significant relationship between entrepreneurial enthusiasm and professional misconduct.[36]

Ninety-four percent of the pharmacists in Quinney's sample agreed that "the public expects the pharmacist to be both a business man and a professional man." On the basis of various questions about professional values, Quinney concluded that about 45 percent of his sample were attuned to both roles, while 16 percent were more oriented to a professional than to a business role, 20 percent favored the business side, and 20 percent were indifferent, adhering to neither position. Among the pharmacists with a business orientation, 75 percent were law violators; in contrast, none of the pharmacists favoring the professional role had been cited for a prescription violation. In the middle, 14 percent of the pharmacists attuned to both roles, and 20 percent of the indifferent pharmacists were violators. Formal controls, particularly legal codes related to the practice of pharmacy, Quinney concluded, "are made effective by the operation of informal controls (in terms of role expectations) which come mainly from within the occupation." He speculated that his findings might be applicable to the practice of "independent general medicine" because it too manifests the trait of a split professional-business structure.[37]

Although persuasive—in part because it meshes with common understanding—Quinney's study is only a one-shot post facto inquiry. We cannot be sure whether the business attitudes held by the lawbreaking pharmacists preceded their misconduct or followed it, as a kind of cynical defense after the offenders' trouble with the law. Nor does the study take account of differences in personality, age, type of business, and other such factors that affect attitudes toward one's work and toward the law. There is also no satisfactory independent check on whether what the respondents said about being engaged primarily in a business or a profession reflects their true feelings. In matters other than the prescription violations, those with an expressed business orientation may behave more professionally than those who define themselves as professional. We lack satisfactory information about other violations, have no data on the sites of the businesses—whether in ghettos or elite neighborhoods—or the practitioners' incomes, and we do not know whether the owners or their employees were the violators. All these matters could influence our understanding of lawbreaking by pharmacists.

Nonetheless, Quinney's study reveals the two conflicting pressures on professionals who also operate as merchants: the ideal of duty and selflessness versus the desire for gain and self-interest. That some pharmacists, lawyers, and doctors feather their fiscal nests by flouting their professional obligations can undoubtedly be traced to the temptations and opportunities to do so, as well as to the weaker hold of professional standards on them.

THE STUDY OF
WHITE-COLLAR CRIME

The study of white-collar crime, the scholarly arena in which inquiry about matters such as criminal fraud by physicians has been carried on, has been an ungainly enterprise, typically marked by an uneven combination of "objective" social science and indignant muckraking. As John Braithwaite pointed out in a comprehensive review of the field, "White-collar crime research marks a rare case of sociological scholarship having a substantial impact on public policy and public opinion."[38] "Substantial" may be too strong, but research by academics and practitioners, from the muckraking period forward, has undoubtedly contributed to various reform movements, such as those concerned with pure food and drugs, bribery, safety for coal miners, and political campaign contributions.

The term *white-collar crime* was coined by Edwin H. Sutherland in his presidential address to the American Sociological Society in 1939.[39] Sutherland's address mixed moral indignation with scientific research. Ten years later, in a mixture no more distilled, he published *White-Collar Crime*, in which he defined his topic "approximately" as "crime committed by a person of respectability and high social status in the course of his occupation."[40] Several generations of scholars have grappled with the implications and shortcomings of this definition, which does not correspond to legal definitions of criminal behavior. Moreover, under Sutherland's definition, only violators of a certain social status are to be considered white-collar criminals. Nevertheless, Sutherland's term has been translated into numerous foreign languages and is readily understood throughout most of the industrialized world as a shorthand expression for a category of lawbreakers whose occupational crimes-for-profit pose particular concerns.

As a propaganda weapon, the phrase is pithy and pointed. To abandon it because of its imprecision might impede forms of scientific inquiry that have flourished since Watergate and the movements for more recognition of the rights of groups such as blacks, women, and gays. Abandonment would also likely enlarge the gap between social science and popular thought, a gap already widening as social science becomes more quantitative and as it rides its Marxist steed on a national track increasingly dominated by conservative mudders. To adopt staider terms in place of "white-collar crime" ("economic crime," "occupational crime," or "abuse of power") would not solve the problem of imprecision. For our purposes, we will attempt to anchor and nourish our material on medical fraud with insights from the research and theoretical literature on white-collar crime.

Sutherland mentioned medical doctors only once in his 1949 monograph: "In the medical profession, which is used here as an example because it is probably less criminal than other professions, are found illegal sales of alcohol and narcotics, abortion, illegal services to underworld criminals, fraudulent reports and testimony in accident cases, extreme instances of unnecessary treatment and surgical operations, fake specialists, restriction of competition, and fee-splitting." Only fee-splitting comes in for further explication. The fee-splitting physician, Sutherland explained, sends his patients to the surgeon who will pay the largest referral fee, rather than to the one who will do the best work; and, typically, the less skilled the surgeon, the higher the kickback he must give in order to get business. Thus split-fee cases gravitate to the highest bidders, the most dangerous surgeons. Although the practice is illegal in many states and a violation of the conditions of admission to the medical profession in all states, Sutherland estimated that in areas where fee-splitting is rampant, kickbacks range as high as 60 and 70 percent. He also noted, without citation, that two-thirds of the surgeons in New York had been reported to split fees and that more than half of the physicians in a central western state who answered a questionnaire on this point favored fee-splitting.[41]

Sutherland's assumption that the medical profession is "probably less criminal than other professions" is one we encountered frequently during our research. We have no reason to doubt that most physicians are honest, but some of our research, presented in the following chapters, leads us to suspect that doctors who work largely with Medicaid patients are, as a group, probably less honest than other doctors. Our interviews with private insurers suggest that they, too, are often victimized by physicians. There is also some evidence that many doctors who cheat Medicaid also cheat on their tax returns. Of the 11,000 doctors who received $25,000 or more from Medicaid in 1968, for example, more than a third failed to report "a substantial amount" of their income to the Internal Revenue Service; in some instances, the unreported income exceeded $100,000.[42]

That Sutherland chose briefly to explicate only the topic of fee-splitting may reflect the dearth of his material on medical violations and, more likely, his overriding interest in other matters. His comments on fee-splitting contain the germ of an idea that we will carry further. Doctors, as he points out, disagree with the criminal code's condemnation of fee-splitting. This introduces a condition generally not found in traditional criminal behavior: few burglars would argue that burglary should be legal or that burglary is in the best interests of its victims. Doctors' refusal to grant the legitimacy of the criminal code may represent their principled differences of opinion or their insensitivity to considerations the authorities have deemed superordinate, but on some occasions it appears to be little more than a rationalization to excuse their misconduct.

On Sutherland's list of physicians' offenses, only fee-splitting and unnecessary surgery appear with some regularity among the charges government investigators make against doctors today. If performed intentionally, unnecessary surgery can be regarded as equivalent to assault—that is, as a crime that involves not only the theft of money but also personal injury, even death.[43] In the 1970s researchers at Cornell University concluded that at least 10 percent of the 20 million operations then performed annually in the United States were unwarranted. The Cornell survey estimated the annual cost of unnecessary surgery at $3.92 billion. A later investigation found that the rate of surgery performed on the poor and near-poor—financed by Medicaid— was twice that for the general population. The disparity was even greater for some forms of elective surgery to treat conditions that are not life-threatening.[44] An article in the *Journal of the American Medical Association* in 1988 reported that 44 percent of heart bypass surgeries may not be medically appropriate; these patients might have been as well or better off with a drug regimen. One-third of the 85,000 carotid artery operations—a costly and dangerous procedure—performed each year were found to be inappropriate, and another third of uncertain value to the patient.[45] A Ralph Nader–affiliated Health Research Group, after reviewing published studies, declared that "well over 200,000 Americans are injured or killed each year as a result of negligence by doctors."[46]

In a 1984 court case a California ophthalmologist was convicted of performing unnecessary cataract surgeries on Medicaid patients. Over five years, he had bilked the program for a million dollars. A fifty-seven-year-old woman was totally blinded when he operated needlessly on her one sighted eye. When his patients had private insurance or were well-off, he performed the surgery skillfully and successfully; patients dependent on benefit programs were dealt with in a slipshod fashion. He told his Medicaid patients, primarily older Latinos, that cataracts were contagious, and he operated even when he knew the patients did not have cataracts. The judge, in sentencing the doctor to four years in prison and a substantial fine, was particularly critical of other physicians who had appealed for leniency for the defendant. "It's astounding how they could write these letters," he said. "They seem to think the whole trial is a contrivance by the attorney general's office." Then the judge emphasized what had particularly upset him: "In not one of the letters has there been one word of sympathy for the true victims in this case, the uneducated, Spanish-speaking people, some of whom will never see a sunrise or a sunset again."[47]

Some researchers argue that unnecessary surgeries contribute to the higher death rate among people under age sixty-five.[48] The rate of elective surgeries per capita is twice as high in the United States as it is in other industrialized Western countries. It also has been estimated that 90 percent of the tonsillectomies done in this country are not needed and that these operations claim more than sixty lives each year.[49]

Referrals that are not essential, rather than those in which a fee is split, are also common among allegations made against Medicaid providers. Unnecessary referrals are particularly likely to occur when incorporated medical groups include both general practitioners and specialists who share the group's proceeds.

DOCTORS, NARCOTICS,
AND ABORTIONS

Sutherland's other categories constitute offenses in which physicians collaborated with patients, for example, in dispensing narcotics, writing phony accident reports, or tendering illegal medical services. The history of physicians' involvement in two of these offenses—narcotics violations and illegal abortion—provides a backdrop for understanding recent structural changes in the practice of medicine that have affected how and how much doctors violate the law.

Narcotics Offenses

Before World War I doctors legally prescribed narcotic concoctions for a variety of physical and psychosomatic ailments. When narcotics such as heroin were outlawed in 1914, some doctors funneled them to underworld dealers and lower-class addicts, and a few physicians also furnished them to wealthy patients.[50]

The key provision of the Harrison Act of 1919 required physicians prescribing designated drugs to register with the federal government. Enforcement was assigned to the Bureau of Internal Revenue in the Treasury Department. The act was written as tax legislation, a small charge affixed to drugs to improve record keeping. Because the law allowed the drugs to be provided to patients in the course of the "legitimate practice of medicine" and in "good faith," most medical practitioners assumed that "if simple record requirements were obeyed, the federal government should be fully satisfied." Doctors also believed that the "otherwise annoying record keeping would strengthen the medical profession's control of these potent medications."[51]

The doctors were in for a considerable surprise. The regulations issued by the Treasury Department placed tight controls on the prescription of the designated drugs. Complaints from physicians began to appear. A Montana doctor, for instance, wrote the attorney general that "the revenue agents who are neither lawyers nor physicians tell me that [my] prescriptions are in excessive amounts." This early triumph of law enforcement over medicine may be seen as a portent of the fate of medical autonomy under Medicare: "What had been a respectable viewpoint by 1915, although not the dominant attitude of the public— the value of addict maintenance by physicians or others—by 1919 and 1920 had come to seem a great danger and folly. Advocacy of main-tenance was repressed as sternly as socialism. Vigorous protests from a few physicians, congressmen, politicians, and laymen were completely ineffective in modifying legal opposition to supplying drugs for the pleasure or comfort of addicts." In short, the Harrison Act was enforced as a law to protect the nation from the ravages of addiction. Its structure as a tax measure was regarded as an acceptable ruse to attain a moral end by means of a legal fiction.[52]

The most notorious narcotics crimes perpetrated by physicians involved their use of professional access to drugs to commit murder. Dr. Harvey Crippen, for instance, killed his wife with a hyoscine overdose and then surgically dissected her body. Dr. J. Bodkin Adams arguably used his medical skill in the administration of drugs to kill off elderly women after he persuaded them to name him in their wills. Cesare Lombroso, generally regarded as the father of criminology and himself a physician, had noted near the turn of the century that "homicide with the aim of getting the benefit of life insurance is an example of a new form of crime committed by some physicians and favored . . . by new advances in scientific knowledge."[53]

What is particularly notable about doctors and narcotics, though, is the extraordinary and hasty retreat of U.S. medical practitioners from the field once the government began to regulate it. In England, on the contrary, doctors refused to abdicate what they deemed as their responsibility for persons addicted to drugs, and heroin remains legal there today. In the United States, there were a few prosecutions of doctors who defied or tried to evade the authority of the government, and the matter was settled. American doctors had found drug clients largely unsavory, the financial return uncertain, and the whole business not worth the trouble.

Today only fringe practitioners bother with drug traffic, sometimes combining their narcotics infractions with exploitation of the Medicaid program: "He . . . walked three blocks to visit a doctor on Bleeker Street. The doctor's 'office' was equipped with a desk, a chair, a stack of Medicaid forms, and a prescription pad. He handed the doctor his Medicaid card. The doctor wrote down that he had just given Pete a complete physical, four X-rays, a blood test, a urine-sugar test, and a test for venereal disease. . . . 'I'll take 300 Valium,' Pete said after signing the form."[54] In Los Angeles, investigators reported a Medicaid doctor who saw so many patients daily that red, blue, and yellow lines had been painted on his office floor to expedite traffic. Each color represented a different kind of pill.[55]

Abortion

The story of physicians' involvement in the performance of abortions is more complicated. St. Augustine established early Christian dogma on abortion with his fourth-century pronouncement that the soul was not present until the time of fetal quickening; therefore, abortion did not constitute the destruction of a human life prior to that time. In the thirteenth century, Thomas Aquinas placed the initial presence of the soul at the same time as Aristotle had: forty days after conception for a male and eighty days for a female, numbers based on the time that genital development had been discerned in spontaneously aborted fetuses of each gender.

Not until the seventeenth century did the Roman Catholic church take its current theological stand against abortion. Nonetheless, abortions were widely available in the United States. The primary practitioners of abortion at the time were midwives and herbalists, and they advertised their services in newspapers.[56] In the mid-nineteenth century, however, the medical profession launched a crusade to drive the midwives out of business, branding them as immoral and incompetent, as part of its effort to extend physicians' monopoly over medical service. The campaign was marked by a basic contradiction rooted in self-interest: Doctors maintained that abortion was morally wrong but also that only they could determine when it was necessary.[57] "To recapture what it considered to be its ancient and rightful place among society's policymakers and savants," organized medicine adopted a "messianic tone"—one spokesperson proclaimed that "the hospital was a temple in which presided a god"—and portrayed physicians as disciples of "missionary work."[58] The campaign succeeded, and between 1850 and 1900 many states enacted laws that allowed abortions to be performed only when the pregnancy threatened a woman's life, and then only by a medical doctor.

One historian, noting that most physicians at the time believed that abortion was morally unacceptable, comments, "The fact that this belief coincided nicely with their professional self-interest is no reason to accuse physicians of hypocrisy on the issue; instead, the convergence probably helps to explain the intensity of their commitment to the cause."[59] Although hypocrisy may not be a fair charge, doctors did deploy their professional power to force midwives out of performing abortions and to restrict the number of women who received abortions. For now a woman could obtain a legal abortion only if a doctor deemed it necessary.

Doctors soon found themselves with patients who wanted abortions but did not meet the legal standard. This group included teenagers, unmarried women, women with "too many" children, and women who for personal reasons (such as a job or an unhappy marriage) did not wish to bear or raise a child. Women who had the wherewithal and the proper connections were given legal, allegedly "therapeutic," abortions; the less fortunate were forced to resort to back-alley operators, who sometimes botched the illegal surgeries so badly that their patients died.[60]

Between 1939 and 1964, according to one estimate, about one of every five pregnancies in the United States was terminated by an illegal abortion—about one million criminal abortions a year—and at least five thousand women died each year as a direct result of such abortions.[61] Most of the criminal abortions were performed on married women with children; many were performed by licensed medical doctors. Frederick J. Taussig, an authority on abortion, stated that he knew of "no other instances in history in which there had been such frank and universal disregard for a criminal law."[62]

A prominent motivation for doctors who performed illegal abortions was "the desire to obtain a good deal of money without much effort." One doctor, an honors graduate from medical school, admitted that he had made several hundred thousand tax-free dollars in almost a decade by performing illegal abortions: "I decided to do a few abortions in order to get a few thousand [dollars] together and open up a nice office in a good neighborhood," he told the probation officer. "I always intended to quit but somehow I never did."[63]

In 1973 the U.S. Supreme Court in *Roe v. Wade* (410 U.S. 113 [1973]) cited a woman's right to privacy and legalized abortions performed by a physician during the first trimester of a woman's pregnancy. A companion decision, *Doe v. Bolton* (410 U.S. 179 [1973]), declared that physicians had the right to determine whether to perform an abortion. In *Doe*, Justice Blackmun reflected common wisdom when, in a bit of dicta, he wrote, "The good physician—despite the presence of rascals in the medical profession, as in all others, we trust that most physicians are 'good'—will have a sympathy and an understanding for the pregnant patient." (As we shall see, "rascals" is rather a benign circumlocution.)

The relegalization of abortion produced telling divisions within the world of medicine. Within five years after *Roe*, 75 percent of the more than one million abortions performed annually in the United States were done not by private doctors working in hospitals or in their surgeries but in 250 of the country's 500 abortion clinics.[64] Some gynecologists and obstetricians refused to perform abortions because they had moral objections to the procedure. Many did not want to gain a reputation among colleagues or in the community as abortionists. Other doctors resented being put into a position in which patients could treat physicians as mere providers of a service on demand.[65]

With abortion as with narcotics, the medical profession in England more than held its own against the law and the courts, in this case largely by blending the interests of women patients with those of the profession. A stringent prohibition against abortion was enacted in 1803 (Lord Ellenborough's Act), but physicians often ignored its dictates, and their actions in turn were ignored by law enforcement agencies. There was also a thriving abortion business among irregulars, a situation that impelled the *Medical Times Gazette* in 1860 to lament, "Society may talk as much as it likes of free trade in medicine, may patronize herbalists, bone-setters, uncertified midwives, joint-rubbers, pill-makers, and nostrum vendors of all kinds. But it may be assured that in so doing it is nourishing a serpent in its heart, whose venomous fangs are ever ready to dart poison of some kind into its circulating current, not the least deadly of which is the practice of procuring abortion, . . . a practice which is getting to infect this land in so virulent a manner as must soon call for some direct interference by the Legislature."[66]

In a test case in 1938, the English courts legitimized physicians' control of abortion and ruled that medical doctors could rely on their professional judgment without interference.[67] The case, *Rex v. Bourne* (1 Kings Bench 472 [1938]), involved a fourteen-year-old girl who had been raped by two soldiers and become pregnant. Dr. Bourne, a London surgeon, performed an abortion and informed the authorities, asking for a trial that would clarify the law. At trial Bourne testified that the birth of the child probably would have destroyed the young girl's physical and mental health.

The judge noted that Bourne had acted "as a member of the profession devoted to the alleviation of human suffering," and he forcefully led the jury to acquit Bourne with his summation observation: "I think that . . . if the doctor is of the opinion, on reasonable grounds and with adequate knowledge, that the probable consequence of the continuance of the pregnancy will be to make the woman a physical and mental wreck, the jury are quite entitled to take the view that the doctor, who, in these circumstances, and in that honest belief, operates, is operating for the purpose of preserving the life of the woman."

The Abortion Act of 1967 sought to restrict abortions in Britain to a limited number of conditions associated with the pregnancy. The vagueness of some terms in the act, however, was largely a response to doctors' insistence that "too great a degree of precision might enable the pregnant woman to diagnose herself as qualifying for termination and demand the procedure." At the same time, the looseness of the definition permitted many physicians, particularly those not working in the National Health Service, to interpret its provisions very broadly; and the authorities were unwilling to interfere with this exercise of professional power. In Britain, thus, the doctors prevailed, both keeping the courts out of what they regarded as their professional realm and retaining for themselves a monopoly on how to deal with what they defined as a purely medical matter.[68]

With regard to narcotics and abortion, then, the record indicates that in the United States, unlike in Britain, doctors abandoned to the law and the courts what legitimately might be regarded as arenas where they could claim strong professional preeminence. In both instances, having driven nonphysician competitors from the field, some American doctors proceeded to violate the law on behalf of selected patients. These examples are instructive, supporting the tentative generalization that in crucial confrontations with government authorities regarding patients' concerns and physicians' self-interest, organized medicine in the United States has largely looked out only for itself. We will return to this theme later, in our discussion of criminal behavior by doctors in the Medicare and Medicaid programs.

PREMEDICAL AND
MEDICAL TRAINING

Doctors do not train for crime in the way that juvenile delinquents do. Physicians overwhelmingly have been raised in that segment of society that avoids involvement with the criminal law. If their premedical education is to be faulted, a major criticism would have to be that aspiring doctors are so single-mindedly tracked into required technical courses that they do not have sufficient exposure to what are presumed to be humanizing kinds of academic curricula. The manner in which physicians are trained may provide a structural context that paves the way for future deviance and lawbreaking. Students vying for grades in order to attend medical school may resort to deceptive behavior because of the stringent standards demanded by admissions committees. Some premedical students may view cheating on exams as a necessary evil; others may become disinclined to help their colleagues with their class work, since they are in direct competition for a limited number of medical school openings. Such extreme rivalries can lead to callousness and cynicism. Sociologists Howard Becker and Blanche Geer have documented the growth of cynicism and the "fate of idealism" in medical school: "The cynic cuts corners with a feeling of inevitability while the idealist goes down fighting."[69]

The formal education of physicians is believed to exert an important influence on their values in later years, and medical schools are often blamed for failing to indoctrinate students with a strong code of ethics and a decent set of social and political convictions. The possible consequences of this failure extend far beyond the individual doctor's personal shortcomings:

The medically uninformed patient is not in a position to pass sound judgment upon the normative adequacy of what the physician does. Medically informed colleagues are not in a position to know what is being done. These structural facts, therefore, put a special premium on having the values and norms instilled in the student during the course of professional socialization in the medical school. If this is not thoroughly achieved under the optimum conditions provided by the medical school, it is unlikely that it will occur under the often less favorable circumstances of private practice.[70]

Leonard Eron reports on a study of the effect of medical education on cynicism, humanitarianism, and anxiety. The cynic is more likely than his colleagues to agree with statements such as "The law is often the refuge of slick operations" and "I think most people would lie to get ahead" and may be more prone to violate the rules regulating Medicaid. The humanitarian affirms remarks such as "When I hear about the suffering of a particular individual or group, I want very much to help"; such an individual may be less likely to steal from a program that assists the indigent. Eron found that students became more cynical and less humanitarian during their four years in medical school. Fifty-five students' cynicism scores increased over that period, whereas only eighteen students' scores declined. The results on the humanitarian scale were only slightly less discouraging. Forty-five students' scores decreased, and twenty-three students scored higher. The results were taken as evidence "of the homogenizing or leveling effect of the medical school experience," since there was less variance among the scores of seniors than those of freshmen. Similar findings have been reported by others.[71]

Students' cynicism, according to Eron, may be caused by individual psychopathology. He notes that students with the highest anxiety scores were also the most cynical. Anxiety, however, cannot be attributed solely to individual psychopathology. The competitive atmosphere of medical school and the need for high academic performance are obvious sources of stress and anxiety. Anxiety may also grow as medical students become increasingly alienated from friends and family, who no longer share the same experiences and cannot be relied on for advice. In addition, a fear of stigma may prevent the student from seeking the help of colleagues.[72]

The rigors of medical school also may promote alienation among future physicians and increase the possibility of fraudulent behavior by lowering physicians' social interaction with the general population. A Stanford University professor has indicated that students there find premeds "narrow, aggressive, anxiety-ridden, unfriendly, and dishonest."[73] Alienation has been found to be related to criminal behavior. Cressey, for example, reported that the embezzlers he interviewed in prison had, prior to their offense, a "nonsharable" problem, a difficult situation they felt unable to discuss with others.[74]

Those who treat a large Medicaid population also may become more cynical than doctors with more affluent patients. Attitudes about such a clientele are likely to be acquired during medical school, where a large portion of the patients will be indigent. A survey of medical residents in family practice programs in Ohio indicated that, as a group, the residents believed poor patients were harder to deal with and more likely to be late or miss appointments without telephoning.[75] During training, young physicians develop a conception of ideal patients—their socio-economic characteristics, their acceptance of the physician's authority, their personal characteristics—and become interested in "the effect of the patient on the physician's career (income, reputation, development of further skill, fulfillment of his self-concept as a physician)."[76] The dark side of this view comes across pointedly in a statement by an obstetrician-gynecologist working in a metropolitan hospital in California:

I like patients who are intelligent, responsible people, and I hate patients who are irresponsible slobs. The Medi-Cal [Medicaid] patients—the people on welfare—are the worst of the bunch. Since the government is paying for it, they just don't care about what's going on. They don't show up for appointments, and they never call to tell you. They don't take their medicine. They call you Saturday night, three in the morning, with a problem that could have been taken care of on Wednesday afternoon.

On top of that they have very unrealistic expectations . . . wild ideas about what medicine can accomplish. They come in thinking that the doctor waves his magic wand and you get cured. . . . Half of the problems these people have could have been avoided by just minimal precautions—abortions, infections, venereal diseases and all their complications. It's irritating to have to take care of people when they don't make the slightest effort to take care of themselves.[77]

Although Becker and Geer argue that medical students' attitudes are largely acquired from the student subculture rather than from the faculty, they grant that the students learn "the rudiments of the culture of the medical profession."[78] Others have maintained that during their education and training, medical students adopt a professional image.[79] Haas and Shaffir describe the process: "As students move through the program they are converted to the new culture and gradually adopt those symbols which represent the profession and its generally accepted truths. These symbols (language, tools, clothing, and demeanor) establish, identify and separate the bearer from outsiders, particularly client and paraprofessional audiences."[80]

The goal of the medical school socialization process is to produce an individual graced with "autonomy, judgment, skills, commitment, and motivation." Many students may be painfully aware that they are not the superhumans required by the professional model, but there is evidence that they nonetheless begin to play the part of the professional in their interactions with others. Such behavior seems essential to cope with the daily situations that confront the neophytes. Students, for example, assume a "cloak of competence" to mask their uncertainty when dealing with faculty and particularly with patients, who may resent or fear the pretend doctors.[81] Such skills can prove useful to a physician later confronted by investigators demanding explanations for questionable dealings. The "cloak of competence" can be donned to assure the "outsiders" that everything is under control and that whatever momentarily seems wrong can readily be put right.

Students also learn to "medicalize" problems, including those of professional misconduct. There exists "a medical model of social control which views problem doctors as nonculpable and best identified and rehabilitated by medical professionals."[82] Those who have not undergone the long and esoteric training of medical school, the profession maintains, are incapable of judging physicians. This position is learned during medical school: "As students observe and experience the problems of medical care and practice, they develop an understanding and identification with the profession and the ways its members confront their problems. Students are less quick to voice criticisms of what they see, as they come to take the role, directly or indirectly, of those they will soon follow."[83]

Physicians are likely to judge the errors of their colleagues in "normative" terms—that is, as something any physician might do given the circumstances.[84] These attitudes inhibit doctors from reporting the wrongdoing of colleagues to authorities and from testifying against other practitioners. This view also informs the profession's response to the punishment of deviant doctors. The establishment of impaired physician programs by state medical societies to rehabilitate errant colleagues is evidence of the institutionalization of this philosophy; state licensing boards, rather than taking official actions, often allow doctors to join these programs.

CORRUPT CONDUCT

A recurring theme in this book centers on the debate over whether physicians' misconduct is caused mainly by systemic influences that create deviant doctors or whether the blame for medical criminals rests primarily with individuals. The literature we have presented thus far suggests that the medical school is partially culpable for the creation of medical students' eventual illegal behaviors. Much of this literature, however, follows Parsons's structural functionalist theory of human institutions.[85] Such an approach supports the view that the medical school is "a well-coordinated institution performing its primary function effectively. . . . Insofar as there were problems in 'socializing' students to the expected role, these derived from the different abilities or personalities of individual students rather than from any fundamental deficiencies in the schools themselves."[86]

Individual pathology among medical practitioners may be at the root of some misconduct and fraud. About 20 to 40 percent of medical students are said to need psychological help, but it is unclear to what extent medical school is responsible for their problems. Some argue that a major source of maladaptation in medical school is the individual's personality prior to admission; others maintain that medical school admission committees fail to screen candidates adequately in terms of potential problems.[87]

Common sense suggests that greediness plays a role in billing scams, but there are no hard statistics to show that doctors today are more avaricious than their predecessors. A director of pediatrics residency at a large hospital, however, had no doubts that younger doctors were increasingly motivated by money and power:

Because of my personal background and my professional feelings, I still put in sixty to eighty hours a week. But I have a very difficult time finding responsible people who feel the same way I do to help me take care of my patients. By my standards, most practicing physicians and young physicians in training—regardless of what the new youth are saying—are primarily interested in ripping off the public and getting power. . . . Twenty years ago, I would have one, two, at the most three people whom I would consider avariciously motivated monsters. This group is now five to ten times larger than it used to be—comprising 25 to 30 percent of the trainees. These people are taking advantage of the system, of their colleagues, of the nurses that work with them, and of their patients.[88]

Results of a survey of individuals involved with medical education also suggest that economics has been having more of an impact on students' attitudes as applicants increasingly come from high-income backgrounds. Opportunities for high incomes, however, have always played a strong role in decisions to enter medicine.[89]

Nonetheless, the recent growth in physicians' incomes and concomitant business responsibilities is unprecedented. Doctors in training, however, rarely learn much about the business side of the work they will do. Their instructors, university-based professors, tend to be too removed from the routines of everyday practice to offer useful guidelines. Moreover, medical students learn to distance themselves from the cares of their patients, fearing that emotional involvement would make their work intolerably depressing. Such distancing can facilitate exploitation, particularly when the victim is not a human being but an impersonal government bureaucracy, such as Medicaid. (It has become a truism of criminology that offenders are more readily able to carry out monetary crimes after defining their victims as large, heartless institutions, easily able to absorb financial losses.)[90]

Medical students may also learn that their professional status permits them to get away with nonmedical wrongdoing, that their aberrancies will be overlooked or treated indulgently: "Medics, especially in countries where they begin their training as undergraduates, are often the most rowdy, bawdy and irresponsible of all students, and such behavior, which would be considered outrageous in others, is indulged or condoned."[91]

Besides this, medical students often assume large personal debts to finance their education and training. Students graduating in 1987 had an average debt of $37,732.[92] Efforts to repay these loans may push new doctors toward unacceptable financial tactics when they begin to practice.

Attitudes regarding medical benefit programs are inculcated early in the training of future doctors. A survey of 144 medical students enrolled at the University of California, Irvine, found that most third- and fourth-year students regarded Medicaid in the same unflattering light as did practicing physicians. They rated the program particularly poorly in regard to administrative dimensions such as efficiency, reimbursement rates, and cost-effectiveness. (Students just beginning their schooling were much more likely to respond "don't know" to questions about Medicaid.) When asked about the causes of fraud and abuse against Medicaid, 35 percent of the students blamed the nature of the program, not the nature of the violators. Only 1 of the 144 students suggested that better medical education, with a stronger focus on ethics, might help reduce fraud.[93]

The way in which physicians come to engage in criminal acts against Medicaid accords with the thesis of David Matza, who in a classic monograph, *Delinquency and Drift*, emphasized that juvenile delinquents do not *always* violate the law, though this lesser part of what they do comes to overwhelm all other aspects of their behavior. The delinquent, Matza notes, "drifts" between illegal and conforming behavior. Similarly, physicians who cheat government programs are virtually never committed to a life of crime and, indeed, may cheat on only a small fraction of their billings. Matza explains the notion of "drift" as it applies to juvenile delinquents in the following terms: "Drift stands midway between freedom and control. Its basis is an area of the social structure in which control has been loosened. . . . The delinquent transiently exists in limbo between convention and crime, responding in turn to the demands of each, flirting now with one, now with the other, but postponing commitment, evading decision."[94]

The drift into delinquency is a gradual process, often unperceived by the actor. The first stage may be accidental or unpredictable from the point of view of any attempt at theoretical explanation. Matza describes the "situation of apprehension" for delinquents with a scenario that corresponds closely to that for many Medicaid fraud cases. He points out that if delinquents were really committed to lawbreaking behavior, there would be little shame or guilt when they are captured. Like the doctors in our study, Matza's delinquents agree that someone should be apprehended and punished for misdeeds, but it ought to have been someone else. At the same time, in language that bears remembering as our stories of physician fraud unfold, Matza notes of the delinquent: "He excuses himself, but his gruff manner has obscured the fundamental sense in which he begs our pardon."[95]

Ideas such as these will recur in our analysis of lawbreaking by physicians directed against the Medicaid program. The "subculture" of medical delinquency, as we will document, includes a wide range of behaviors. Some doctors cheat regularly, some nudge gently beyond the tolerable limits of government regulations, and many on occasion merely do what they want, knowing that they should not but thoroughly confident, as well they might be, that they will never be caught. Minor violations tend to be written off as a function of the tension between government regulation and standard professional norms. The uncertainty of so many medical situations—stemming from the fact that the practice of medicine is an inexact science and a form of art in which there are legitimate differences of opinion about the same set of symptoms—allows physicians to rationalize minor lawbreaking acts. Doctors' behaviors that result in trouble with the law tend to be of an egregious nature. Although we will pay most attention to such matters, it must be remembered that, like much of white-collar crime, the acts of apprehended physicians undoubtedly represent no more than the tip of the conning tower of a very large and very elusive submarine.

Chapter Two

Medicaid and Medicaid Fraud

The social problem posed by Medicaid fraud has not yet reached the center stage of public concern, even though abuse of the system threatens the health and well-being of millions of Americans. But many aspects of Medicaid fraud are both too complex and too mundane to grab headlines or present network photo opportunities. Moreover, few instances of fraud are notorious enough to command attention beyond the communities in which the malefactors practice. Thus, although the sum total of Medicaid violations constitutes a considerable drain on the health, financial resources, and integrity of our nation, none of the cases prosecuted to date have turned Medicaid abuse into a prominent social issue.

One impediment to a grass-roots crusade against Medicaid fraud is surely the fact that the principal victims—the poor—do not routinely command great shows of respect or sympathy. Another obstacle to public outcry for reform is that Medicaid fraud can be depicted as a peripheral issue to the far more serious problem of how to provide adequate medical services for all Americans. Energy and attention devoted to antifraud efforts can be regarded as energy and attention that might better be concentrated on reaching a nationwide political consensus about plans to improve the delivery of medical care. In this context, overutilization of services, the core of fraud and abuse, can be seen as no more than a distraction from the major concern: the underavailability of health care in the United States.

Claims are sometimes made that those who concentrate on Medicaid fraud play directly into the hands of those who want no real structural changes in what remains an inadequate approach to health care delivery. Focusing on fraud can be compared to adopting the tactics of a faltering political regime: start a war against another nation in order to divert attention from domestic disarray and thereby resuscitate internal support. This line of argument possesses a good deal of validity. Accusations that unconscionably greedy doctors are bleeding the national exchequer can (and do) compete with reports seeking to demonstrate that the reach of benefit programs is severely inadequate. If fraud were ignored, perhaps programs would expand more rapidly.

Our contention, however, is that although attention to fraud is ultimately of less significance than the availability of quality health care, the two issues are interrelated. In our concluding chapter, we will consider ways to reduce fraud *and* improve medical care.

1976—REDEFINING THE MEDICAID PROGRAM

From the start, Medicare possessed considerably greater public appeal than Medicaid. So, for roughly the first ten years of its existence, Medicaid had to struggle to gain a firm foothold within the federal and state bureaucracies. During Medicaid's second decade, there was much gross and fine tuning of the program, as state and territorial jurisdictions sought to fashion a satisfactory health care delivery system for the indigent. By the start of President Reagan's first term, however, the focus had shifted away from concerns with extending health care services to an intense interest in oversight and cost containment. Despite Reagan's ideological hostility to government health benefit programs, however, no effort was made to dismantle Medicaid. The program had become too important to too many people for either major political party to discuss eliminating it.

The first major exposé of Medicaid fraud came in 1973, when William Sherman, a reporter for the *New York Daily News*, wrote a twelve-part series of articles based on personal visits on the city's Lower East Side to what became known as Medicaid "mills." Sherman posed as a Medicaid beneficiary seeking treatment. Typical is his report on a visit to a podiatrist.

The patient was ushered into a small room on the second floor where a young receptionist took his Medicaid card, began filling out an invoice, and then said, "We are going to X ray your feet." "But I want to see the podiatrist," insisted the patient. "He's busy; go into that room for X rays," she insisted. "You haven't asked me what is wrong yet; nobody has even seen my feet," he argued. "It doesn't matter," she said. "The city requires that we X ray everybody's feet before we see them." The patient refused and a health department podiatrist said later that it is absolutely ridiculous to X ray someone's feet before you examine them. More importantly, it is unhealthy to expose someone to radiation unnecessarily.[1]

The podiatrist at this facility was the highest biller of the 702 doctors in that subspecialty practicing in the city. He was often seeing more than fifty patients a day, though health department authorities insisted that thirty-five is the maximum any podiatrist can handle daily and still provide quality care. The Medicaid mill podiatrist also had billed for sixty toe jackets at $11.20 apiece during a single day of practice; the average podiatrist rarely makes more than four jackets on any day. (Toe jackets are made of moleskin from a plaster cast of a toe and fit over the toe like a miniature sock. They are used to protect an arthritic or deformed toe.) When some of the podiatrist's patients complained that their toe jackets collapsed in a few weeks, it was discovered that he was using polyfoam instead of moleskin. On the basis of this complaint, the podiatrist agreed to make restitution of $6,000 to Medicaid and to undergo a short suspension from participation in the program.[2]

Sherman's Pulitzer prize–winning investigative report undoubtedly inspired a similar enterprise several years later, again in New York City, by Senator Frank Moss (Dem.-Utah), the chairman of the Subcommittee on Long-Term Care of the Senate's Special Committee on Aging. On a June morning in 1976, Moss, wearing shabby clothing and armed with a Medicaid card bearing his name and the address of the Statler Hilton Hotel in New York, presented himself at the East Harlem Medical Center for treatment of a "cold." Later in the day, he used the same approach at the 164th Street Clinic in the Bronx. Both visits led to blood and urine tests, follow-up appointments, and prescriptions that were to be filled at pharmacies adjacent to the clinics. The East Harlem Medical Center also gave Moss a chest X ray and referred him to a chiropractor.[3]

In an election year, Moss's theatrics caught the fancy of the media. David Mathews, secretary for the Department of Health, Education and Welfare (HEW), denounced Moss's performance as "grandstanding," no more than a cheap attempt to embarrass the Ford administration. Mathews was said to have told a cabinet meeting that his office was well ahead of Moss in identifying the problem and solving it. Indeed, six months earlier, Mathews had announced an audit of the states with the largest Medicaid programs and those individual practitioners who treated large numbers of Medicaid patients. John Walsh, a former FBI agent, had been named the first director of the Office of Investigations, a newly established 74-member criminal arm of HEW,[4] and a Medicaid fraud-and-abuse unit of 108 agents had been created in HEW to help the states identify and prosecute cases of fraud and to establish more effective management systems. These actions, valuable to blunt the force of Moss's message, had come in response to the disclosure during Senate hearings a year earlier that the government had but one part-time employee dealing with Medicaid fraud and abuse.

Indeed, by 1976, Medicaid had become a political hot potato. Both Congress and the administration wanted to contain the rapidly escalating program costs but did not want to bear any responsibility for denying medical services to needy people. Tough rhetoric against abuse and fraud seemed a way of avoiding that fundamental impasse.

The earliest sensational stories about Medicaid fraud had focused on "welfare queens" who were allegedly bleeding the benefit programs, but these exposés soon gave way to analyses showing that crooked providers were responsible for far more losses than were errant beneficiaries. Management chicanery also surfaced. Charles Cobbler, who had held high-level positions in various HEW bureaus dealing with Medicaid, was forced to resign when it was disclosed that he had been getting kickbacks from companies for having helped them gain Medicaid fraud-control contracts. Moss's subcommittee concluded that Medicaid was "not only inefficient, but riddled with fraud and abuse" and recommended that additional federal funds be allocated for enforcement. Meanwhile, Senator James Buckley, a conservative Republican from New York, was urging that the health budget be slashed $1 billion "to crack down hard on health-care crime."[5] By Buckley's logic, the sheer size of the Medicaid budget lent itself to fraud; a slimmer slice would permit better oversight.

Most notably, no one at this time was proclaiming that the real national challenge was to ensure that Americans not yet eligible for Medicaid were granted coverage and to provide better, more comprehensive services. The talk of reform rested squarely on cost containment, and the national mood grew parsimonious in spirit: Each of us best look out for ourself, and let the devil take the hindmost. The notion that illness is fortuitous was under political challenge, which, in turn, suggested a more tightfisted response to claims for more munificent redistributive programs. Other concerns, particularly those connected with national defense, had replaced welfare priorities. It had become anathema—politically suicidal—to call for increased taxes to redistribute wealth from those who had a great deal to those who had less than a decent share: Budgets were to be balanced by cutting expenditures. The Reagan administration's success in reducing inflation, slicing interest rates, and raising the level of employment offered dramatic testimony to the apparent efficacy of this approach. That these economic achievements came at the cost of a wildly out-of-control national deficit remained arguable and less compelling than the tangible results of the turnaround for those who had not been left behind.

LEGISLATING HEALTH CARE

Medicaid had come into existence along with the other Great Society programs maneuvered through Congress by Lyndon Johnson's administration. In the health benefit programs cost considerations were subordinated to the goal of providing essential services to the nation's most vulnerable populations, the poor and the aged. The anticipated cost of the medical benefit programs, though high, was not regarded as intolerable.

What was highly problematic at the outset, though, was whether the

proposed programs could secure the support—or at least the acquies-
cence—of the medical profession. The American Medical Association
(AMA) had been mounting heavily funded efforts since the 1940s to
lobby against any discussion of federal programs that admitted any hint
of national health insurance, which most physicians considered tan-
tamount to the "enslavement of the medical profession."[6]

The AMA wanted to extend private health insurance, such as Blue
Cross, while keeping the government as far away from the medical
business as possible. Inaugurated in the 1930s, Blue Cross and Blue
Shield were fee-for-service programs whose fees were determined by
local boards and committees. Physicians had a board majority in about
two-thirds of the nation's seventy-odd Blue Shield organizations and
controlled the fee-review committees in virtually all of them. Surgeons
are said to have dominated the Blue Shield movement. Allegedly, they
saw to it that fees for operations were generous. (Later, when Medicaid
came along, it simply adopted the surgeon-favoring Blue Shield pattern.) By the 1960s Blue Cross and Blue Shield plans provided medical
coverage to about 40 percent of the employed population (ranging from
6 percent in Nevada to 91 percent in Rhode Island).[7]

The unemployed almost invariably had no medical benefits. The
elderly, because they did not make good insurance risks, found it
particularly difficult to enroll in medical insurance plans. The insurance industry, in a critical break with the AMA, welcomed the idea of
federal medical support for the elderly, believing that its members
"would be relieved of an obligation to extend their insurance carrier
functions." The AMA argued against any program in which eligibility
was based on age alone, insisting that government health insurance
should be administered on a local basis and that recipients should have
to be needy.[8]

The AMA mounted a ferocious campaign against the passage of
health benefit legislation, aiming its guns almost exclusively at Medicare, casting the fight as "an all-out battle" brought on by the Johnson
administration throwing down "the gauntlet" and "challenging organized medicine." To get out its message and defeat Medicare, the AMA
spent a million dollars both in 1964 and 1965.[9]

Lyndon Johnson's landslide victory in the 1964 presidential race provided the climate for passage of the medical benefit program package the following year. Wilbur Mills, the Democratic chairman of the House Ways and Means Committee, a powerful force favoring the legislation, realigned the committee's membership in accord with his party's electoral sweep, assuring a favorable reception of the three-part bill he then introduced to create the federally supported medical programs.

The major part of the legislative package, which was to become Medicare coverage for Social Security beneficiaries, reflected a Senate subcommittee report that three-quarters of older Americans lacked adequate hospital insurance. Also included, almost as an afterthought, was a plan to cover the medical expenses of the indigent. Costs of this latter program were to be paid from both state and federal funds, though administration would reside with the states and state participation would be optional. The blueprint that became Medicaid was built upon the existing federally enacted Kerr-Mills program, which had been approved by the AMA, whose president declared that its retention was integral to "our long fight to guarantee future generations of Americans the blessings of a progressive and dynamic system of medicine, unhampered by government control." Kerr-Mills, however, was regarded as a "general disaster" because only a few wealthier states had participated in the voluntary program. Medicaid, seen as nothing essentially new, largely escaped the fire of the AMA.[10] The organization correctly understood that the program would not affect the power elite of the medical profession, but might provide more business for its marginal members.

Congressional debate, media comment, and AMA lobbying focused on the ideological premises of the benefit programs, but Johnson's mandate, combined with his extraordinary knowledge of the means to maneuver measures through Congress, led to the enactment of Medicare and Medicaid in 1965. Medicare and Medicaid became Title XVIII and Title XIX, respectively, of the Social Security Act (24 U.S.C. 1396). Medicaid eligibility was offered to indigent persons who were disabled, blind, over sixty-five years old, or members of families receiving welfare aid for dependent children. States were permitted to expand their programs, if they chose, to include a "medically needy" or "spend down" group (persons within the four specified categories whose income was above the eligibility limit to qualify for welfare). Such individuals paid "deductible" sums based upon their monthly income.

Each state also was free to increase or to contract the services it offered under its Medicaid program. Some of the additional services would be subsidized with federal funds; others would not. The states also retained the right to determine eligibility for Medicaid and to set payment procedures and expenditure levels. The federal legislation, however, demanded basic coverage of a minimum of seven services: inpatient and outpatient hospital care, physician's services, laboratory work, X rays, nursing home costs, family planning services, and periodic screening, diagnosis, and treatment for children.

Today all states have Medicaid programs. Arizona and Alaska, the last to do so, inaugurated them in the 1980s. For a time, Arizona had claimed that the medical needs of its Native American population would impose an intolerable fiscal burden on the state budget, and Alaska had made the same claim about its Inuit population. In 1982 the federal government began to reduce its share of contributions to Medicaid but exempted states that met at least one of these three conditions: (1) operation by a state of a qualified hospital cost review program, (2) an unemployment rate in a state exceeding 150 percent of the national average, and (3) demonstration of certain levels of financial recovery through programs for controlling fraud and abuse.[11]

In at least one respect, Medicaid can lay claim to some success: It appears to have improved the health of its clientele. A careful analysis concluded, "Considerable progress was made in selected areas of health that have traditionally been poor for low-income people and that are amenable to medical care—infant mortality rates . . . and deaths from pneumonia and influenza, cervical cancer, cerebrovascular diseases, diabetes mellitus, and accidents."[12]

The growth of Medicaid has coincided with—and perhaps influenced—a dramatic reduction in the country's neonatal mortality rate (the number of deaths of children under twenty-eight days of age). The neonatal mortality rate has declined notably since 1970, according to the National Center for Health Statistics, and dropped 6 percent between 1989 and 1990. But glaring discrepancies persist between whites and blacks: The gap in infant mortality between whites and blacks has continued to grow, and the U.S. infant mortality rate lags behind that of twenty-one other nations. Japan's infant mortality rate, for instance, is less than half that of the United States.[13]

Despite evidence of the improvements in the health of Medicaid beneficiaries, a few lonely voices insisted that the program did not do nearly enough. Congressman Claude Pepper, for instance, used to argue that the program largely provided "sick care" rather than health care, noting that it focused on crisis intervention, rather than on keeping healthy people healthy.[14]

IGNORING FRAUD AND ABUSE

The original Medicaid blueprint did not much attend to questions of fraud and abuse. The guidelines in regard to these matters, set forth in section 1902(a)(w), declare that states must "provide . . . such methods of administration . . . as are found by the secretary to be necessary for the proper and efficient operation of the plan." It would be some time before this vague provision was translated into specific oversight policies. The statute did include a provision for sanctions against those who violated the rules: "Whoever for the purposes of causing an increase in any payment authorized to be made under this title, or for the purpose of causing any payment to be made where no payment is authorized under this title . . . shall be fined not more than $1000 or imprisoned for not more than one year, or both."[15]

The possibility of widespread fraud and abuse apparently was not seriously considered either in the drafting of the legislation or in the congressional hearings and debates concerning it. For one thing, there had been little warning from the private insurance companies, such as Blue Cross, that abuse would be a significant matter. That private insurers did not raise this alarm can be explained in two ways. First, as programs based on actuarial calculations, systems such as Blue Cross were only passingly concerned about rising expenses due to fraud and abuse because premiums could readily be adjusted to cover payments. Second, a large segment of the private insurance field was controlled by the medical profession, whose members had been chronically un-interested in carefully monitoring the business behavior of colleagues.

More important, sponsors of the new legislation were wary of arous-ing new waves of antagonism from the AMA by implying that physicians were other than scrupulously honest and perfectly capable of keeping their business dealings within the confines of what the law allowed. To have challenged this shibboleth, Congress would have risked escalating an already tense conflict into all-out warfare. Physicians tend to see themselves as a cut above others and as members of a profession that vigorously punishes its wrongdoers.[16] Evidence to the contrary existed, but Congress chose simply to ignore it. In 1961, for instance, the General Accounting Office (GAO) accused physicians who were pro-viding medical care to dependents of armed services personnel of over-charging the federal government $3 to $4 million annually, and in 1965 witnesses before the Senate Antitrust and Monopoly Subcommittee had alleged that "money hungry" eye doctors were using pressure tactics to coerce kickbacks from dispensers of eyeglasses.

Despite such omens, members of the government and Congress turned their backs on the potential for fraud because they feared a wholesale unwillingness on the part of disgruntled physicians to par-ticipate in the benefit programs. The new laws did not require doctors to accept patients for whom the government was paying, and there were many suggestions that doctors would turn away these patients. In 1961, in a statement regarding an early version of Medicare, for instance, the AMA declared that the medical profession "will not be a willing party to implementing any system which we believe to be detrimental to the public welfare." The AMA considered boycotting Medicare but was scared off, in part, by the possibility that such an action would violate the antitrust laws.[17] Fear of physician nonparticipation was so real that President Johnson authorized the use of veterans' hospitals for any elderly person denied treatment under the new Medicare program.

Physicians used the threat of noncooperation to ensure that the final regulations reflected their views. To obtain doctors' allegiance, legis-lators did not incorporate into Medicare a fee schedule for physicians but mandated instead that doctors be paid "their 'usual and customary' fee, provided that the fee was reasonable"—the same payment standard used by the physician-dominated private insurers.[18] Further compromises placed faith in physicians' integrity rather than relying upon outside scrutiny and judgment. In an interview we conducted, an attorney for the AMA offered one example of the way things had gone:

When the law was originally written, it was that he [the physician] had to certify [a need for hospitalization] before the patient got admitted to the hospital, and recertify after a certain length of time so that there would be somebody's signature there authorizing continuing payment of a hospital bill, and we [the AMA] argued that under past procedures . . . the fact that you had admitted a patient to the hospital was considered evidence that you thought he should be in the hospital. This seems reasonable and, for once, a reasonable argument won out, so that the initial certification got dropped from the law, but the recertification was retained.

The fact that many hospitals are owned by doctors and that competition among them was often cutthroat went unattended in the face of medical pressure. Congress accepted the medical profession's portrait of itself as above such grubby tactics as overutilization of hospitals. Doctors, everyone concurred, responded to a higher ethic, and there was no conflict among patient, physician, and government interests.

The federal government ignored fraud and abuse at the inception of the benefit programs also because it needed to establish public confidence in the undertakings. To highlight fraud and abuse might have undermined such confidence. A high-ranking enforcement official whom we interviewed captured the sense of indifference about misdeeds that marked the initial phase of the administration of the medical benefit programs: "It seems as though when all of this originated they said, 'Let there be a program.' They felt they were dealing with a community group that was full of integrity and would not violate the precepts of the program. From 1965 until about 1968 there was no such thing as fraud and abuse."

According to experts, there was plenty of blame to go around. Wilbur Cohen, a Johnson aide, noted that Congress did not enact the controls necessary to prevent fraud and failed to monitor the medical program it had established. The executive branch did not recommend the needed legislative changes, did not use its authority to enforce the law, and did not use its authority to demand that the states enforce the law. States largely abdicated their oversight responsibility, Cohen maintained, and local medical societies also closed their eyes to obvious abuses by members of their profession.

THE PROBLEM OF
GROWING COSTS

"It went so fast," said a person deeply involved in the passage of the early legislation, "that neither [Congressmen Mills or John Byrne, the committee minority leader] worried about costs."[19] But within a few years the rapidly escalating costs of the benefit programs began to make government authorities uneasy. The administration had predicted a price tag of $2.25 billion for 1968, when it was anticipated that forty-eight states would have Medicaid programs. The actual expenditure for that year proved to be $3.54 billion even though only thirty-seven states took part.[20]

Inflation fueled early cost overruns, as did supply and demand. By 1966 the United States was already facing a doctor shortage, and the benefit programs greatly increased. Medical care expenses also rose because services practitioners had previously provided without cost now could be reimbursed by Medicaid and Medicare.[21] Products and services that once had been beyond the means of poor patients came into common use with federal financing. Besides, many physicians increased their prices to take advantage of government reimbursement. Medicare, for instance, had agreed that doctors would get 80 percent of their usual and customary fees; many physicians inflated those base fees to pump up what they would receive.

ENTER FRAUD AND ABUSE

The earliest investigations of fraud and abuse focused on recipients. An HEW audit agency review of the first two years of Medicaid operation in New York charged that "the New York City Department of Social Services has not satisfactorily implemented procedures to identify and proceed against recipients who obtained medical assistance on the basis of fraud and misrepresentation."[22] But it soon became obvious that there were distinct limits on how much an unqualified beneficiary might cheat. For most people, especially those who are reasonably healthy, the illicit quest for free medical services is hardly an appealing enterprise.

By 1967 provider fraud cases were beginning to surface. The first case in California to result in a prison sentence came that year, when a pharmacist in Los Angeles was charged with stealing more than $20,000 from benefit programs. He had behaved with stunningly reckless stupidity, submitting bills during a nine-month period that showed him dispensing more of a particular drug than all the pharmacies in the state dispensed for the entire year. Program monitoring came in for passing mention in the report on the feckless pharmacist: "We are well aware that the present machinery for detecting such abuses is inadequate," declared Charles O'Brien, California's chief deputy attorney general. "I doubt that unless [the pharmacist] had made obvious mistakes he would have been caught for a long time."[23]

Medicaid fraud began to receive federal attention when members of Congress tried to find ways to contain costs. In mid-1969 the Senate Committee on Finance entered the fray with charges against physicians for "gang visits" to hospitals and nursing homes. Doctors, the committee declared, were submitting bills for seeing as many as fifty patients a day in the same facility, regardless of whether the visits were medically necessary or whether any medical service was rendered. In a rapid foray through these sites, a physician could "earn" hundreds of taxpayer dollars at the expense of a few smiles and some small talk. The committee charged that physicians also had begun to bill separately for services that previously had been routinely included in the fee for an office visit. An individual close to the committee said, "Some Congressmen now think it's time to tighten the language of the act to hold down doctors' fees and reduce cost."[24]

In 1970 Lowell Bellin, the first deputy commissioner for New York City's Department of Health, told another Senate subcommittee that the city was planning to examine the records of any physician who made more than $5,000 a year from Medicaid.[25] Both New York City and the state of New York by this time were overwhelmed by the skyrocketing cost of Medicaid, which had increased about 500 percent since its inception and would go up another 400 percent in the following four years. The city's fiscal crisis was intimately tied to welfare expenses, and much of the early battle regarding Medicaid services and fraud control would be fought in the state of New York. The approach to financing Medicaid adopted by the state of New York underlay a considerable part of the problem. In thirty-six states the cost of Medicaid was divided between the state and the federal government, with no requirement for local financial participation. Fourteen states required some sharing of costs between the counties and the state. New York, with its huge Medicaid budget, required counties to foot one-quarter of the bill. New York City was particularly hard hit by the state's financial approach.[26]

These financial woes were aggravated by the New York legislature's decision at the inception of Medicaid to provide all nonmandatory services for which federal matching funds were available. The range of services covered by Medicaid in New York thereby came to exceed that of most private health plans. New York had also added the nonmandated "medically indigent" to its Medicaid rolls, with liberal eligibility requirements. The 2.5 million New York residents eligible for Medicaid at the height of its beneficence put a terrible stress on the budget.

In 1968 and 1969 New York tightened its eligibility requirements, and thousands were removed from the Medicaid rolls. Altering eligibility standards left a sour taste, but tossing unscrupulous providers in jail offered diversionary prospects for politicians. Surprisingly, 1970 congressional hearings on Medicaid abuse by physicians aroused only routine objections from the president of the Medical Society of New York, who reflexively suggested that portraits of fraud were exaggerated and that most doctors were not crooks.[27]

Although eligibility for Medicaid in New York City was determined by the Department of Social Services, the health department established and monitored the standards of care. Under the leadership of Lowell Bellin, a physician, the health department was determined to investigate Medicaid abuses. Bellin started to call himself a "medical cop,"[28] and the AMA lodged protests. Early in 1971 the department audited nonprofessional providers and soon announced that transportation companies had bilked the benefit programs out of millions of dollars. Ambulance services had charged Medicaid for trips taken by patients who had been dead for months and by others who were still hospitalized.[29] In response to the shift away from investigating doctors, the AMA now supported Bellin's efforts at curbing abuse. For his part, Bellin found it far easier to prove cases against ambulance companies than against physicians.

Medicaid violations also were commanding attention from a Manhattan grand jury. Early in 1972 a grand jury report detailed numerous forms of criminal behavior by providers:

Payment for services not rendered, often procured by forging patient signatures or having patients sign Medicaid forms prior to treatment, such as dental work and physical therapy to the elderly. Payments for unauthorized or unnecessary services, such as tooth extractions, x-rays, a bridge, and referral visits to other medical specialists in a Medicaid group. . . . Payments for defective pharmaceutical devices, such as vaporizers and corrective footwear. Payments for brand name drugs when generic name drugs were provided.[30]

The grand jury also faulted the city's administration of Medicaid, arguing it was contributing to the delinquency of providers, and estimated that almost a billion dollars had "gone down the drain" since the program had started. The city was said to have failed to establish patient and provider profiles to detect abusive practices, despite a federal government order to do so. Nor was a system in place to determine multiple payments to providers. The city's failure to pay providers promptly also led some cash-poor practitioners to sign on with "factoring" companies, which bought the receivables and charged providers a 12 to 15 percent commission. The grand jury believed that doctors often inflated their Medicaid claims to recoup the commissions paid to the factoring organizations, which themselves sometimes included phony claims with the real ones. (Factoring was banned in November 1976.) Finally, the records for detection and prosecution of fraud were said to be in such deplorable condition that they were proving useless for the task.[31]

Media attention focused not on the structural deficiencies outlined by the grand jury, but on estimates of the extent of fraud in New York City's Medicaid program. Mayor John Lindsay took umbrage at the grand jury's announcement of a billion-dollar loss, countering with the

claim that the grand jury had found less than $5 million in unautho-
rized charges and that city officials had already identified the culprits
and collected $3.5 million of the specified amount through "regular
procedures." Lindsay insisted that less than 0.2 percent of the Medicaid
bill had been identified as illicit cost and that enforcement was working
just fine. The issue was thus put to rest, and the grand jury report "did
not prompt any agency changes regarding fraud and abuse."[32]

MEDICAID MILLS

"Medicaid has become an unmanageable monster in New York City,
consuming billions of dollars," proclaimed William Sherman in his
series of articles on Medicaid mills in the *New York Daily News* in 1973.
Not to be outdone, competitors of the *News* soon launched their own
investigations of the Medicaid mills.[33] These mills were the most
sensational form of fraud spawned by Medicaid. Located in dilapidated
areas, often in storefronts, and catering almost exclusively to patients
on the Medicaid rolls, the mills resemble clinics in that doctors with
different specialties are gathered under one roof. But the mills' providers
often rent space in the building and bill Medicaid individually. Many
of the mills' doctors are members of ethnic minority groups or foreign
medical school graduates, practitioners who would find it difficult to
establish their practices in affluent white neighborhoods. In 1976 it was
estimated that Medicaid mills accounted for more than 70 percent of
program payments in New York City.[34]

Criminal activities flourished in the Medicaid mills. Some employed
"hawkers" to round up customers. Several catered to drug traffic.
During the four-month congressional subcommittee investigation that
featured Senator Moss's undercover stint, various government agents,
all claiming to be suffering from nothing more ominous than a cold,
had been seen by eighty-five doctors in Medicaid mills. They underwent eighteen electrocardiograms, eight tuberculosis tests, four allergy
tests, as well as hearing, glaucoma, and electroencephalogram tests.
Collectively, they were given seven pairs of glasses without having been
examined by an optometrist. Only one doctor failed to fall for the scam,
telling an investigator: "Get out of here; there's nothing wrong with

you." More typical was the following experience: "His 'head cold' was diagnosed as 'sinusitis,' he was given a general physical, an EKG, told he had a severe heart murmur and that he probably had rheumatic fever as a child. In addition, the doctor ordered a series of X rays of the patient's sinuses and chest, and referred him to a heart specialist—all in the space of three minutes."[35] Other legislative investigators had similar experiences. At a Los Angeles clinic, an agent was told that her urine sample was normal—even though she had turned in a watery soap-and-cleanser concoction.[36]

An official, who asked not to be identified in a news commentary, deplored the Medicaid system of offering unlimited services without controls. He suggested that if Senator Moss or his colleagues had gone to a private specialist in Chevy Chase, Maryland, he might also have received unneeded tests and prescriptions. The difference would be that the senator, not the taxpayer, would pay.[37]

Although Medicaid mills are sometimes staffed by dedicated doctors who choose to work among the poor, more often they are run by practitioners locked out of any other form of medical practice. That Medicaid mill doctors were the first to be charged with fraud reflects their vulnerability and lack of professional power. The Medicaid mill operators were guilty of the charges made against them, but they also were scapegoats for doctors in more fashionable positions who also engaged in abuse.

THE CASE OF DR. MATTHEW:
A WATERGATE FALLOUT

Revelations in 1973 about the illegal acts committed by the Nixon administration as part of the Watergate burglary and coverup helped step up the pace of investigative reporting on other fronts. The case of Dr. Thomas W. Matthew illustrates what happened across the country when journalists began to scrutinize the Medicaid program.

Matthew was arrested in April 1973 and charged with "diverting" $250,000 in Medicaid payments from his Interfaith Hospital, a drug treatment center in a squalid section of Queens, New York. The facility, the district attorney said, was filthy, and neighborhood residents were seeking to have it closed because of the brawling they said it engendered. Early newspaper stories spotlighted Matthew's ties to President Nixon. The doctor frequently had praised Nixon for his support of "black capitalism," and Nixon had pardoned Matthew in 1969 after the doctor served two months of a six-month sentence for income tax evasion.[38]

A decade before his arrest for Medicaid fraud, Matthew reportedly gave up a $100,000-a-year practice as a neurosurgeon to become, according to the *New York Times*, "an inexhaustible activist with the zeal of a country preacher and the vocabulary of a scholar." Matthew opened the Interfaith Hospital in 1964 and soon thereafter organized a black self-help group with the acronym NEGRO (National Economic Growth and Reconstruction Organization). In 1966 Matthew met Richard Nixon, and a few years later President Nixon instructed government agencies to provide "all assistance possible" to the doctor. Matthew ultimately got $8.2 million from Medicaid for building his hospital, $2.4 million in defense contracts, $400,000 in bonds, a $227,000 loan from the Small Business Administration (SBA), and $20,000 from the Office of Economic Opportunity.[39]

The discovery that Matthew had diverted funds from Interfaith Hospital led the state to remove the hospital's Medicaid certification and downgrade Interfaith to a "health-related facility"—a rank below a nursing home.[40] The investigation also discovered that the city had incorrectly advanced Interfaith $1,228,545.

Matthew had used the Medicaid monies to help NEGRO projects. He claimed that these projects—a bus company in the Watts area in Los Angeles and a New York City factory—had provided employment for Interfaith's recovering addicts and therefore were part of the treatment. The prosecutor argued that no proof had been offered to substantiate this claim and that, even if it were true, such job placement was not part of the treatment regimen defined by Medicaid.[41] Matthew also was charged with using grant money to pay his airfare and that of twenty aides on a trip to the Soviet Union.

Matthew was found guilty of seventy-one counts of illegal use of Medicaid funds and given a three-year prison sentence—a price he said he regarded as payment "for being a pioneer." Before he was sentenced, further details of his relations with the Nixon White House surfaced.

The SBA had looked into Matthew's activities after he defaulted on his loans, but a House subcommittee investigator told the committee that "the White House tried to get the Small Business Administration to burn its files" on the doctor. The SBA auditor added that his boss had told him to "get rid of the report."[42] Instead, the investigator had forwarded his findings to the Department of Justice, which tried to recover $175,000 from the doctor. The subcommittee was also told that the White House had refused to furnish the Queens district attorney with reports on Matthew; the district attorney was convinced this denial was intended to prevent additional political embarrassment.

Medicaid fraud was not confined to Republicans. Dr. Louis Cella, the leading contributor to the Democratic party in California, was tried and convicted of thirty-two felony counts. Cella padded hospital bills by $12 million to cover his political contributions, and he failed to file tax returns for three years. Eventually he served thirty-two months in a federal prison for his fraudulent activities. On release, Cella went to work in a rural clinic in Coachella, California, that primarily serves migrant farm laborers. His office wall was adorned only by pictures of Cesar Chavez and Robert Kennedy. Of his prison experience, Cella said, "It's a Greek tragedy in which everyone dies."[43]

Watergate proved to be a catalyst. Before it, scrutiny of Medicaid was perfunctory or nonexistent; after it, some of the protective cover that had hidden the wayward activities of powerful persons and groups was stripped away.[44] Watergate produced an atmosphere ripe for reform in which liberal members of Congress could move much more forcefully to fashion and enforce laws against Medicaid fraud.

When the Democrats regained the White House in the fall 1976 elections, the reform-minded Carter administration moved into previously taboo areas. In a random audit of providers, the federal government found that only one of fifty-three doctors had no discrepancies in the twenty-five claims examined for each doctor. The government also released for the first time the names of doctors and others convicted of defrauding Medicaid. Joseph A. Califano, Jr., secretary of Health and Human Services, hoped making names public "would serve as a strong deterrent to those relatively few physicians and other providers who seek to line their pockets with taxpayers' hard-earned dollars."[45]

PSROS—A FAILURE IN
PROFESSIONAL SELF-REVIEW

Attempts to control untoward actions by powerful constituencies typically first focus on self-regulation. The wayward group argues that a few bad apples had escaped attention but that, alerted to the danger, the group will monitor and cleanse itself. Such a stance is difficult to counter because there is likely to be no substantial evidence that it is self-serving; besides, any challenge would imply a lack of confidence in the integrity of the group and its ability to fulfill the duty it vows to undertake. Those under siege also traditionally claim that only they have the specialized knowledge and wisdom necessary to comprehend and solve any problems in their ranks. More ominous is the implicit threat that if the group does not have its way in regard to self-regulation, it will make it very difficult for outside enforcers to carry out their work.

In 1972 the annual bill for Medicaid had soared to $7.35 billion, and Congress, frantically looking for some way to constrain costs, authorized the establishment of Professional Standards Review Organizations (PSROs), a plan for self-review by the medical community. The initial mission of the PSROs was to monitor the care and costs of services being delivered to hospitalized Medicare patients. Later, the purview of the PSROs was supposed to be extended to Medicaid, but the patent insufficiency of PSROs as control mechanisms soon became evident and the planned expansion was dropped. The PSROs merit attention here because they represent an example of an approach often advocated to control fraud and abuse in government medical benefit programs.

By establishing the PSROs, Congress intended to remedy a critical gap in oversight that had been addressed in hearings in the late 1960s before the Senate Finance Committee. In many parts of the United States, Medicare patients were admitted to hospitals without any pre-admission review. Because hospital costs represented the largest category of program expenses, any cuts in the length of patients' hospital stays would lead to sizable decreases in program budgets. The issue obviously was loaded with danger: One or more sensational cases of patients dying after having been denied hospital admission or having been released prematurely would surely create a public uproar.

The PSROs were established by the Social Security Act Amendments of 1972 (Public Law 92-603). The same law increased the maximum fine for fraudulent acts against Medicaid and Medicare from $1,000 to $5,000, though the maximum prison term remained one year. To make it easier for prosecutors to prove their cases, the law specified that it was illegal for anyone to furnish items or services in the benefit programs in return for a kickback, bribe, or rebate. The PSRO reflected Congress's twin concerns with costs and care: "Services for which payment will be made . . . will conform to appropriate professional standards for the provision of health care and . . . payment for such services will be made only when, and to the extent medically necessary." PSROs were to develop norms for diagnosis and treatment based on practice patterns in each PSRO region. These norms were to be applied to prospective, concurrent, and retrospective review of institutions, practitioners, and patients.

The legislation stipulated that the individuals who were to conduct these reviews would be physicians, not government watchdogs.[46] Self-regulation was deemed appropriate, given that medical services usually cannot be evaluated by outcomes easily recognized by laypersons; typically, physicians are the only persons truly qualified to evaluate medical services. Thus, Congress accepted the medical profession's claims for exemption from outside scrutiny. But the physicians overlooked a much tougher axiom of political life: Those who pay the bill call the shots. Legislators were willing to be generous to the AMA, which after all was a major campaign contributor, but should voters become dissatisfied, politicians would dump the AMA before losing an election over Medicaid costs.

The PSROs were a way station along the road of decreasing congressional receptivity to the medical profession's claims for hands-off treatment. That Congress was beginning to balk is evident in the stipulation that a doctor's participation in a PSRO could not be contingent upon membership in a county or state medical society.

The PSRO program outraged the AMA, which found it an invasion of professional autonomy: "PSRO poses a greater threat to the private practice of medicine than anything ever developed by Congress," declared Malcolm Todd, then president-elect of the AMA. But Todd thought it best to get inside the tent and urged that doctors work with the new program. Organized medicine feared that even stricter regulatory schemes might be in the offing if doctors boycotted the PSROs: "The failure of PSRO," wrote two experts, "may well initiate other, less workable forms of bureaucratic control over the practice of medicine."[47]

The PSROs, however, proved unable to do what Congress intended—to spot blatant abuses without slashing needed services. One reason for this failure was the decision to limit PSRO activity to reviewing hospitals. Hospital inpatient billings account for about two-thirds of the government's dollar expenditure for benefit programs, and "inappropriate" hospital utilization may account for 10 to 35 percent of such expenditures.[48] But hospital admissions were already undergoing review because of institutional requirements. Peer pressure, generated by word-of-mouth critiques and gossip in the encapsulated medical world of the hospital, exerted at least a minimum kind of control over blatant abuse. By directing the PSROs to review hospitalization practices, Congress ignored the area under the least scrutiny and likeliest to yield the greatest harvest of abuses: the office practice of medicine.

Peer review also has other shortcomings in the realm of medical practice. It may be true that "peer judgments of the quality of clinical care . . . are neither sufficiently accurate or sufficiently homogeneous to be of practical use in decision making by government or by third-party insurers." It is true that doctors are notoriously unwilling to label the practices of fellow physicians as deviant. As Elliot Freidson's research shows, doctors define aberrant behavior in normative terms; that is, they tend to excuse variations as actions some doctors might reasonably undertake, and they are willing to censure only the most outrageous acts.[49] This overly charitable attitude greatly restricted the cost-cutting potential of hospital peer review, though some doctors might well have avoided recommending admissions to avoid PSRO oversight.

The effectiveness of the PSROs was also inhibited by the virtual identity of the regulators and the regulated—that is, community physicians were supposed to pass judgment on other physicians from the same community. This and other structural difficulties greatly hindered the PSROs:

PSROs must begin with a core of local physician support—one or more highly intelligent, articulate physicians committed to peer review in general and to the PSRO variant of it in particular, and respected by local colleagues. Physicians with all these qualities are not in abundant supply, and physicians with the respect of their colleagues who are willing to risk leadership into controversial areas are especially few. These physicians (assuming their presence) must then increase their numbers to constitute a board of directors to work to develop the organization, instead of (as some boards have) using their control to make sure that it does little or nothing. They must then "sell" their PSRO to their peers, who are often indifferent, sometimes hostile. They must then show a keen eye for managerial talent in selecting an executive director, who must himself display the rarely combined skills of technocrat (for data-related tasks), diplomat (in dealing with doctors and hospitals), and manager (in running the organization from day to day).[50]

Another factor that prevented the PSROs from achieving the twin goals set by Congress was that the goals themselves—better care at lower cost—were unrealistic given the course of contemporary medicine, which is based on ordering more tests and using more expensive equipment. Previously untreated maladies, such as hypertension, eating disorders, sports injuries, and substance addiction were receiving increased attention as reimbursement under both public and private programs became available. PSROs could hardly fault such developments.

The PSROs also erected a barrier between themselves and the law enforcement agents. In an interview we conducted, a disgruntled investigator described his experiences:

The unfortunate part about the PSRO—some PSROs are really effective, but then again—those that were successful and effective got run out of town. The unsuccessful ones were the kingpins of the local AMA.

I had severe problems with a couple of PSROs. They didn't even want to give me records. I say, "Wait a minute. We pay you. What the hell are you talking about—you won't give me records? You're working for the federal government." All this was sacrosanct information, this information on patients.

Congress empowered the PSROs to punish offending physicians by refusing Medicaid payments for unacceptable treatment and by excluding doctors from participation in the benefit program. But only rarely did PSROs resort to such measures; instead, they preferred educational efforts such as informal meetings, small conferences, bulletins, and explanations of guidelines. During the eleven-year experiment with peer review boards, from 1973 to 1984, the PSROs formally disciplined a total of seventy hospitals and physicians.[51] The government was less than satisfied with this particular venture into self-regulation by the medical profession.

CRIMINAL ENFORCEMENT
EFFORTS

Up through the mid-1970s the states had done little on their own toward policing fraud and abuse in Medicaid. A congressional staff report pinpointed the structural difficulty that had undercut state interest in enforcement: "The fundamental underlying problem is that Medicaid is a bifurcated program in which the federal government pays most of the money but leaves enforcement and program efforts to the states. The states have been happy to accept federal funds but not the responsibility to police Medicaid."[52] Hearings in the U.S. House of Representatives in 1975 found that twenty states had not audited a single Medicaid provider or referred anyone for prosecution during the time the program had been in operation—almost a decade for some of the states. For example, when the Los Angeles District Attorney's Office sought to create a Medicaid fraud unit, the county board of supervisors, according to one of our interviews, vetoed the proposal because so little local money was involved in supporting the program.

In 1976 Congress belatedly established the first full-time federal position to oversee the enforcement of Medicaid programs (Public Law 94-505). The Office of Inspector General (OIG) in the Department of Health, Education and Welfare was charged with seeking out fraud in any of the HEW-financed programs and recommending corrective action concerning "fraud and other serious problems."[53]

The following year the Medicare and Medicaid Anti-Fraud and Abuse Amendments of 1977 were passed in response to congressional review of abuses. The amendments upgraded program violations from misdemeanors to felonies (thereby increasing the maximum prison terms and fines), required more explicit disclosure of ownership and control of health care organizations, improved the professional standards review program, implemented internal administrative reforms, and provided technical revisions to clarify existing rules.[54] Senator Herman Talmadge, who introduced the bill, said it provided "an opportunity to send a clear, loud signal to the thieves and the crooks and the abusers that we mean to call a halt to the exploitation of the public and the public purse."[55]

The amendments also sought to clamp down on kickbacks to doctors by expanding the definition of wrongdoing to include any remuneration that sought to induce the referral of Medicaid or Medicare patients. In New Jersey, Medicaid investigators had found laboratories making direct cash payments (called "greens") to doctors; providing personnel paid for by the laboratories but working for the doctors; "renting" space in doctors' offices; and providing goods and services, such as surgical supplies and cigarettes, to doctors. A laboratory manager in Monterey Park, California, later testified that, in his experience, kickback arrangements were "rampant" and that of the ten thousand doctors in his area, "as many as a couple thousand are rotten."[56]

In addition to enacting the Anti-Fraud and Abuse Amendments, Congress passed legislation requiring each state to establish a Medicaid Fraud Control Unit (MFCU) within the state attorney general's office or another office that had criminal prosecuting authority (Public Law 95-142). The law also required that the MFCUs be separate and distinct from the single-state agencies that administered Medicaid. The MFCUs were to have the capability to investigate potential Medicaid fraud and the ability to prosecute cases or formally refer cases for prosecution; they were to develop procedures to review complaints of alleged abuse and neglect of patients in health care facilities receiving payments under the state Medicaid plan and, where appropriate, to act on such complaints or refer them to appropriate state agencies for action; and they were to provide for the collection or referral to an appropriate agency for collection of overpayments made under the Medicaid plan.

At first, agency rivalries hindered the work of the MFCUs. Initial investigative leads could come only from the Medicaid agencies in the states, which had previously been responsible for policing the program. They resented having to yield this function and often disliked having to share (or lose) headlines that resulted from a well-publicized enforcement action. Cooperation between the state agencies and the MFCUs was slow to develop; later the MFCUs began to generate their own caseloads. State agencies also feared that uncovering fraud would undermine public confidence and physician support of the program.

The enforcement situation improved for the MFCUs in 1982, when federal oversight responsibility for them was transferred from the Health Care Financing Administration (HCFA) to the OIG in the newly christened Department of Health and Human Services (HHS). The OIG, charged by President Reagan to be "as mean as a junkyard dog," took a much more supportive stand toward the MFCUs than the service-oriented HCFA.[57]

By 1989 thirty-nine states and the District of Columbia had MFCUs. Most states with the highest Medicaid costs created MFCUs, but only three of the ten states with the lowest Medicaid expenditures have such units. The nonconforming states have claimed that there were too few violations to justify creating a separate, new enforcement agency or that they wanted to retain their fraud-control work within the state Medicaid agency and were perfectly capable of handling the problem.[58] The House Select Committee on Aging remained unpersuaded by these explanations and cited more invidious considerations. The committee believed that states had not applied for 90 percent federal funding mainly because of the resistance of state Medicaid administrators, who did not want to share their powers or have them taken away from them. According to the committee, political jealousies had interfered with the establishment of a viable network and a national commitment to detect and prosecute those who committed Medicaid fraud.[59]

MFCU administrators often maintain that their work is judged not by the importance of the cases they deal with but by the amount of money they recover. It was not by coincidence that New York City started up an investigative unit for medical benefit program fraud when the city was facing a severe fiscal crisis. The focus on repayment, rather than justice, forms the basis of the lament of one MFCU chief, who told us in an interview: "As a prosecutor I am not a revenue-producing system. There are ethical problems with the whole concept of prosecution for profit. We are strictly a criminal adjudication function. The federal government—those agencies in the federal government that have monitored us—namely HHS and Congress—don't share my sensitivity in that regard and feel that we should be a revenue-producing operation."

THE 1980s:
MORE COST CONTAINMENT

By the 1980s government officials viewed the medical benefit programs as a decent idea gone wildly astray. The health bill shot up 15.1 percent in 1981, easily outpacing the 8.9 percent inflation rate. The cost of the programs made the early euphoria about providing adequate health care to all Americans seem like a distant, wry, and anachronistic fantasy. Medicare, though, had achieved a sacrosanct aura—and attracted a large, vocal, and powerful political lobby. In contrast, Medicaid was quite vulnerable to political pressure, although the federal government, which had the power to mandate structural changes in the programs, had a far smaller financial interest in Medicaid than in Medicare.[60]

But some states felt they were sinking under the weight of out-of-control costs for Medicaid. In 1979 the lieutenant governor of California called Medi-Cal "a medical monster, in danger of becoming a self-service vending machine dispensing billions of dollars to the health industry."[61] And so the California legislature led the way in 1982 by introducing radical structural changes in Medicaid as it sought to bring a large budget deficit into line. Medicaid had always permitted recipients to use the doctor or hospital of their choice, as long as the provider accepted Medicaid. Now the state legislature empowered Medi-Cal and private insurance companies to offer their business to providers who agreed to charge less than the competition. A Medi-Cal "czar" was named to negotiate contracts with hospitals.[62] The hospitals now had to agree to treat patients for flat per diem payments instead of the fee-for-service billing to which they had been accustomed. Another dose of competition was injected into California when Blue Cross, with the legislature's authorization, began "preferred provider" coverage. Under its terms, clients who visited specified providers were excused from having to make copayments.

The state's $400 million worth of Medi-Cal cuts (from a budget of $5 billion) included the elimination of payments for codeine compounds and other pain relievers and decongestants. To compensate, aspirin was added to the list of drugs for which payment became available under Medi-Cal. Payments to doctors and hospitals were reduced by about 10 percent. Three hundred thousand medically indigent Californians—adults between twenty-one and sixty-five who were so poor they would have been forced onto welfare rolls if they had to pay their own medical costs—had their care turned over to the counties, which were given 70 percent of the money the state had been spending on their care. Governor Jerry Brown defended the changes by insisting that the "whole concept is to put the state in the position of being a prudent buyer instead of having to pay whatever it is charged." A former health director for the state took another view, calling the changes "a totally thoughtless, mindless exercise in bureaucratic terror, designed to frighten people away from seeking care."[63]

Two years later, a study published in the *New England Journal of Medicine* reported that 4 indigent patients had died and the conditions of 182 others had worsened after the California legislature had taken away their Medi-Cal benefits. Expanding on this study, the same authors found that lack of access to treatment or uncoordinated medical care had contributed to at least four of the seven deaths among medically indigent adults during the year; in a control group whose members did not lose their insurance, there was only one death and it was not related to the quality of care.[64]

In a 1989 court ruling, a California judge decreed that when Medi-Cal had decided to stop paying for a patient's oxygen, it should have given the patient ten days' notice before cutting off her benefits and should have continued benefits during her appeal. The judge stated that "cost consciousness must not take precedent over the legitimate medical needs of the recipient for continued services."[65] But his was a weak voice amid a cacophony of cries for cost containment.

DIAGNOSTICALLY RELATED
GROUPS (DRGs)

The federal government, wary of so dramatic a move as California's, instead sought to rein in Medicare costs by instituting a payment program based on diagnostically related groups (DRGs). Like PSROs, DRGs were planned eventually to cover Medicaid, and some Medicaid fraud cases were discovered through their use. Under the DRG approach, the state, rather than the hospital, was to set a price for hospital services based on a patient's diagnosis, which was to be coded into one of 467 DRG categories. Since hospitals would not be reimbursed in excess of the preestablished price, they would have to control their costs in order to prosper financially.

Partly as a result of DRGs, in 1984, for the first time in ten years, the cost of private health care insurance increased only modestly, largely because of a sudden and sharp drop in hospital use.[66] Nonetheless, the DRG system offered numerous opportunities for provider abuse:

Concern has been raised over the possibility of providers attempting to maximize profits through such tactics as reducing the level and quality of care given to a patient, inappropriately shifting patients from inpatient to outpatient status, and prematurely discharging and then re-admitting complex cases under a higher-paying DRG assignment. . . . Since a DRG system sets compensation by diagnosis made, there is a natural tendency for a provider to look at the patient's total bill and to find an appropriate diagnosis which will cover the incurred costs, or even cover and give an additional profit. . . . A hospital may determine that under the DRG program, certain types of patients can be treated at far lower prices than paid by the state. This may cause a hospital to over-advertise these services and encourage patients and doctors to over-admit patients with that diagnosis. . . . Hospitals and doctors may encourage certain kinds of unnecessary treatment while at the same time refusing to perform certain tests or procedures because they do not generate a healthy profit.[67]

Fearing that the medical profession could not be trusted—out of either concern for patients or self-interest—to follow the new guidelines strictly, Congress next created Peer Review Organizations (PROs) to serve as watchdogs for the DRG system. Unlike the failed PSROs, the PROs were to be private companies that hired physicians to evaluate health care–related practices and determine whether services are reasonable and medically necessary, meet professionally recognized standards, and are provided economically.[68] The PROs were to recommend sanctions to the inspector general of HHS, who would have 120 days to approve or disapprove the recommendations.

The PROs were told to "get aggressive," and three that remained passive were soon terminated.[69] During the first seven and a half months of their existence, PROs began proceedings against 950 doctors and 183 hospitals. Sanctioned physicians were fined and/or suspended from the benefit program and were reported to their state medical boards for possible further sanctions. Up through 1987 the government had approved sixty-five PRO sanctions, mostly against physicians.[70] The power of the PROs was further enhanced by the Health Care Quality Improvement Act, which granted immunity to physicians and hospitals from civil damages in lawsuits brought by physicians dissatisfied with PRO decisions and their consequences.[71]

By 1988 there were fifty-four PROs. Each PRO is supposed to keep detailed data profiles on physicians and hospitals, to create scorecards on those with quality problems, and to intervene with an educational regimen or recommended punishments when scores reach certain levels.[72]

CONCLUSION

The growth of officials' concern about fraud and abuse perpetrated by physicians and other providers in the Medicaid program correlates directly with rapidly escalating government expenditures for health care. There continues to be heated debate about precisely who or what is to blame for the striking increases in the price of health care in America. Doctors' incomes have outpaced inflation by such a great margin that it is extremely difficult to argue they have not seized the opportunity to promote their fiscal self-interest when they can. It can be (and often is) argued that physicians formerly were underpaid, particularly relative to their investment in an arduous course of training and the priceless value of their services. It is also argued that technical advances in medicine and the salary demands of other providers, such as nurses, have contributed to the cost of medical care. New equipment must be purchased to ensure quality patient care; purchasers are then tempted to use the new equipment whenever possible in order to amortize the outlay. And as medical intervention helps people live longer, there are more older people, who inevitably need more medical care.

Despite these technological and demographic realities, the public has viewed the rising cost of medical benefit programs, especially Medicaid, with belligerence and bewilderment. Medicaid's price tag—$1.9 billion in its first year—now stands at $61 billion and is rising rapidly. Three major avenues of reform are available: reducing services, reducing the cost of services, and reducing the financial hemorrhaging caused by fraud and abuse.

Efforts to reduce Medicaid fraud, however, have been at best half-hearted. At times, government has rallied the good apples to support enforcement efforts against those who are contaminating the barrel, but doctors are reluctant to criticize colleagues whose sins are less than egregious. Nonetheless, although Medicaid was designed to improve citizens' access to health care, it has also increased government's regulation of health care providers: "Medicaid not only resulted in medical providers becoming more dependent on government for income, the program has also provided an entree for greater government regulation, assessment and review of their services than in the past. Moreover, the playing of the easy money game by some providers has tended to undermine the claims that the medical profession should regulate its own house."[73]

To date there has been no sustained campaign to mobilize public opinion in a moral crusade against Medicaid cheating. In sociologists' terms, Medicaid abuse has not yet risen to the level of a social problem: "A social problem is not just an objective condition or set of objective conditions, because not all objective conditions, including those which pose a real threat, get defined and treated as problematic within the society."[74]

The legislative architects of Medicaid, for reasons noted earlier, refrained from establishing coherent policies or systems for fraud control in the medical benefit programs.[75] Only in congressional hearings during 1969 and 1970 was provider fraud and abuse defined as a serious problem. In 1972 Congress placed its hopes on PSROs; in 1977, on the state-run MFCUs; in 1986, on PROs. To understand why these enforcement efforts have proved unsuccessful, we now turn to the various obstacles and barriers they have encountered.

Chapter Three

The Law in Action

Enforcement in the Medicaid Program

Four facts about physicians' violations of Medicaid regulations require emphasis. First, the cost has been enormous, and the most significant implication of this siphoning off of Medicaid monies is that it has robbed the government of funds that could have provided adequate medical care for every person in the nation.

Second, fraud diverts time and energy away from patient care. When doctors thrust themselves into sleazy acts, all aspects of their professional lives and personal relationships suffer. A particularly ugly aspect of Medicaid fraud is that many doctors who cheat are already so well off that their depredations become especially unappetizing demonstrations of greed.

Third, the physical harms that ensue from Medicaid fraud are more likely than the fiscal cheating to arouse a level of moral indignation that could lead to public and political support for reform. Significant changes in regulatory regimes typically arise not from systematic analyses of their shortcomings, but in response to dramatic disasters. Take the matter of coal mine safety: the 1941 Mine Inspection Act followed the death of 91 miners in West Virginia; the 1952 Federal Coal Mine Safety Act was passed after an Illinois blast that took 119 lives; and the 1969 Federal Coal Mine and Safety Act was primarily a response to a West Virginia explosion that killed 78 persons.[1] But although often grim, the physical harm resulting from Medicaid violations tends to be hidden. There are no explosions, nobody is trapped in a life-and-death situation underground, there is no vivid drama. Persons may be blinded by unnecessary cataract operations, but the acts are spread over time and there is nothing to be done about them. Reformers typically exploit the high rate of infant mortality in the United States to support their plea for better health care, but aggregate numbers such as those involved in worldwide comparisons of national rates do not pack the kind of punch that moves the populace or those with the power to change existing arrangements.

Fourth, the subtle erosion of confidence, trust, and faith that accompanies the exposure of physicians for malfeasance surely weakens the social fabric. It may be healthy for citizens to realize that doctors are not godlike, but it does not seem desirable to live in a society in which everyone distrusts everyone else. So-called white-collar crime creates widespread suspicion, uneasiness, and cynicism—and provokes law-abiding citizens to wonder if they are stupid for not being on the gravy train.

The low visibility and the low level of public indignation associated with Medicaid violations contribute to a notable fact about enforcement in the Medicaid programs: Few physicians who break the laws are apprehended, prosecuted, or convicted. Of course, public apathy is not the only consideration undermining government enforcement efforts. Doctors are powerful, and their professional associations are diligent in blocking regulatory plans that might imply that the "superior calling" of physicians is just another business or industry.

In order to understand how enforcement works, and why it has failed, we obtained official reports and conducted face-to-face interviews with Medicare and Medicaid officials responsible for the integrity of program operations. We also talked with American Medical Association officials and enforcement agents in Washington, D.C., Illinois, Indiana, New York, Florida, and California, including federal field investigators, staff in the Office of Inspector General and the Health Care Finance Administration of the U.S. Department of Health and Human Services, state prosecutors who handle medical fraud cases, personnel in Medicaid Fraud Control Units, and officials in state-contracted companies ("carriers" or "fiscal intermediaries") who administer payments for the benefit programs. We conducted about sixty interviews, with the average interview lasting about one to two hours. In almost all instances, our respondents were forthcoming. They answered freely and appeared truthful, even giving responses that showed themselves in a poor light. In general, the agents exhibited a certain amount of cynicism about their jobs, doctors, and our project.

DETECTION OF
MEDICAID FRAUD

Attempts to estimate the extent of various kinds of fraud, abuse, and waste in American health care invariably turn up figures that by reasonable standards seem stunningly high. A Medicaid audit of doctors, pharmacies, and medical laboratories in 1977, for instance, found that 90 percent had billing irregularities.[2] It is virtually impossible to determine which portions of such "errors" are attributable to ignorance, sloppiness, or duplicity, but the errors rarely favored the customer. Add to this the common anecdotal evidence of hospital patients who complain of extraordinary charges for aspirin, toothbrushes, and other items—some of which they neither want nor use—and one begins to form a picture of what appears to be ubiquitous waste as well as tactics that likely involve fraud.

Investigations to determine the extent of deception that occurs in ordinary medical practice—as opposed to Medicaid mills—by "shopping" doctors (that is, by using undercover agents posing as actual patients) would face considerable resistance on ethical grounds, including allegations of entrapment and harassment, and objections to the deflection of scarce medical resources from their proper purpose.[3] Nor could investigators easily conclude which services that seemed unnecessary simply represented a legitimate difference in judgment rather than fiscal self-aggrandizement on the part of the provider. Victimization surveys of the general population, which uncover a good deal of traditional crime previously unknown to law enforcement authorities, would not be useful for discovering the extent of medical crime because victims of medical fraud rarely know that they have been bilked or that an injury is the consequence of unnecessary and unwarranted medical procedures. Even if patients were aware of illegal charges, the matter would not be of much concern; bilking insurance companies carries a much different emotional loading than being bilked personally.

Criminal prosecution of physicians suspected of malfeasance is particularly difficult because the state must produce evidence that will pass the "beyond a reasonable doubt" standard. Investigators often express mock amazement that any errant physician is ever apprehended, despite the virtually limitless number of offenses committed. One investigator compared the prevalence of lawbreaking doctors to a grossly overstocked fish pond, where the merest attempt easily nets prey. But the way the system actually works, he pointed out, is that "the only ones we get are the fish that jump into the boat." Only the blatantly indiscreet, seemingly totally disorganized, or astonishingly thoughtless physicians are snared, and they keep the enforcement apparatus sufficiently occupied, the investigator maintains, to allow the rest to proceed unmolested. These "smarter" miscreants routinely victimize the medical benefit programs by ordering unnecessary tests and procedures. Such overutilization is unlikely to be discovered, and if it is, it is considered "abuse" rather than "fraud." "I think if a guy is smart, he'll go with the overutilization because he isn't going to go to jail for it," an investigator noted. Patterns of illegal behavior are hard to detect because most offenders wrap their misdeeds inside the seemingly normal practice of their trade. The very nature of medicine effectively limits the possibility of a physician's being called to task for what he or she has done.

Enforcement agents also point out how insurance rules can tempt doctors into wasteful or unnecessary procedures. For example, since insurance carriers do not reimburse physicians at the going rate for the time spent obtaining a patient's complete medical history, a doctor may truncate such a discussion in favor of blood tests, X rays, electrocardiograms, and similar procedures, which may be either arguably necessary or not necessary at all. Were more money paid for face-to-face talks between physicians and patients—with bills specifying the amount of time involved, in the way that attorneys charge for such services—enforcement agents believe that many, if not most, doctors would spend no more time with patients but would bill for what was allowed.

That doctors tend to charge whatever the reimburser will bear was documented by the General Accounting Office (GAO) in a study of a federal program providing medical care to military dependents. In ten of the fifteen states studied, doctors were told to charge their normal fees, but they were given a schedule showing the maximum they could charge for various medical problems. On 93.5 percent of the bills submitted, these doctors charged the maximum fee. In contrast, in the five states whose doctors had not been given a schedule, only 32.5 percent of the claims reached the maximum level.[4]

Enforcement agencies' limited budgets also play a significant role in restricting the detection and sanctioning of white-collar crimes such as Medicaid fraud. In the words of a high-ranking Medicare enforcement official: "To go after these guys we need an army and all we've got is a battalion, if that." Virtually every investigator we interviewed felt that if he or she had more time and resources to devote to seeking out medical crime, it would readily be found, and in huge amounts. The current enforcement system is underfinanced, despite demonstrations that enforcement investments provide sizable cost-benefit advantages. A congressional committee reported that the MFCUs saved more Medicaid monies in one year than had been spent to fund them over the previous four years.[5]

Within the medical service system, however, there is significant resistance to tough law enforcement. Consider the case of the intermediaries who hold federal and state contracts to pay health care providers for services rendered to benefit program participants. Intermediaries are typically insurance companies such as Blue Cross/Blue Shield. When Medicaid and Medicare began, as noted in chapter 2, it was believed that physicians would be reluctant to participate in the programs if they had to deal directly with the government. The taint of receiving federal checks—the same kind of checks that go to Social Security annuitants and welfare clients—offended physicians. It proved strategically necessary to hire private insurance companies, already experts in such work, to pay the bills for government medical program services. The intermediaries were expected to review the bills, but the compensation they received covered only the costs of processing and paying the bills. No money was earmarked or reimbursed for uncovering fraud or abuse. Lacking any budget or fiscal incentive to scrutinize the requests for payment, the intermediaries limited their efforts to determining that the proper forms had been completed correctly. So, in the early years of Medicare and Medicaid, the intermediaries totally ignored fraud and abuse unless it was outrageous.

In the mid-1970s, in the wake of skyrocketing health care costs, combined with congressional hearings and the glare of media attention, the federal government decided that the intermediaries needed to take action to constrain some of the fraud and abuse in the medical programs, and the federal government required them to designate at least one person, who might have other duties as well, to police violations of laws and regulations. Subsequently, during the Reagan years, budget cuts undermined even this small-scale review. As one federal official told us:

Whenever we work with contractors to try to get them to do something in the program integrity [policing] area, they have always had to use people for whom funds were budgeted someplace else. . . . Now it's even worse. For the current budgets they are told to fund mandatory items first, such as bill processing, and then if they have any money left after that they can do the nonmandatory things which get into medical review, utilization review, the areas that do work for program integrity.

[Utilization review] isn't going to be done because they aren't going to voluntarily take money away from that part of their operation on which they are scored—how good an intermediary or carrier they are has something to do with how quickly they process claims and how much it costs.

Unfortunately, program integrity activities are expensive. They are labor intensive. There are just a certain number of things you can do by computer—mass sorting of data. You finally have to get to the human element, and get into some judgments as to whether there is really a problem, and if there is, how to attack it.

Under the current system, the intermediaries bear the primary responsibility for identifying suspect physicians; the government's enforcement agents rely on referrals from the intermediaries. Their detection work, therefore, becomes vital for apprehending these suspect physicians and, if they are guilty, for punishing them.

As part of their efforts to unearth fraudulent acts by physicians, intermediaries routinely used to inform patients of the bills that health care providers submitted to them for services they claimed to have rendered. As could have been expected, this procedure turned up relatively few complaints. Typically, a bill did reflect services the physician had rendered, and the patient had no way to judge whether those services were necessary or appropriate. If a bill itemized procedures performed while the beneficiary was unconscious, medicated, or otherwise distressed, the patient had no way of knowing whether the services had been rendered. Many patients did not bother to scrutinize the bills, since doing so served no personal purpose, and others found the complex documents incomprehensible. Yet other patients had been enlisted by their doctors into conspiracies against the insurance companies. When doctors offered to write down a more complicated procedure than the one they performed, so that the service would come under the payment program or be reimbursed at a higher rate, only an unusual patient might object to such an arrangement.

The intermediaries have discontinued these mailings, and Medicaid patients today rarely see a copy of the bills their doctors submit for reimbursement. This arrangement makes the filing of fraudulent claims that much easier. Worse still, it prevents patients from getting a true sense of the cost of the services and thus protects the medical profession from outraged complaints about exorbitant fees.

In addition to referrals from the intermediaries, enforcement agents get their leads from persons who are privy to incriminating evidence. Only very rarely, however, will a doctor complain about a colleague. Even when patients tell their current psychiatrist about previous episodes of sexual exploitation by other psychiatrists, silence is usually maintained.[6] Several motives are usually proposed to explain the medical profession's notorious self-protective character: practitioners presume that a mark against any physician besmirches them all; practitioners are all vulnerable to allegations of malpractice and therefore must stick together; practitioners have invested so much of themselves to become doctors that they owe allegiance and loyalty to others who have survived the same ordeal.

Recitals of physician's stonewalling in regard to colleagues' tragic mistakes are legion. One example suffices:

Dr. X performed surgery on the leg of a thirty-five-year-old woman. His intention was to tie off the femoral vein. Immediately after surgery, the woman complained of severe pain in the leg, which was noted to be blue and cold, with little pulse. Twenty-four hours after surgery, when there was no improvement . . . , it was realized that Dr. X had mistakenly tied off the femoral artery, not the vein. The woman's leg would now have to be amputated at the hip.

Dr. X . . . was known to have made such errors before, and his surgical privileges had been revoked at a suburban hospital. . . .

Two things interested me. The first was that nobody told the woman anything was amiss. . . . The woman was relatively young, and the mother of two; with one leg amputated, she was now going to have a very different life.

The second was that there was discussion about whether Dr. X would lose his surgical privileges, as if the question were in doubt. (In fact, the hospital did not revoke his privileges entirely. He was merely forbidden to operate alone any longer.)[7]

Much more common than colleague complaints are reports by former office personnel or a disgruntled spouse or lover. About employee informants, one investigator noted, "This happens because the doctor is too cheap to cut them in on the loot. They do the phony stuff for the guy and they're being underpaid. He's cheating them too." With heavy sarcasm, the investigator added, "This tends to breed a certain disloyalty." The same investigator described a different emotional dynamic in cases of patients who have been sexually involved with a physician: "It's jim-dandy for a while, because they are flattered and impressed by it. But after a while they begin to feel cheapened, and when that happens they come in voluntarily. We filed [fraud charges] on one guy and all of a sudden a couple more gals came in and told."

The largest percentage of cases referred to the fraud units, however, are generated by the Medical Management Information System (MMIS), a computer screening process. Ironically, this system itself was conceived in fraud. In exchange for cash and gifts from the companies producing the system, a Department of Health, Education and Welfare official had used his influence to have his agency endorse MMIS and other screening programs.[8]

MMIS calculates various statistics for provider billings, such as the number of patients seen during a working day and the number of services provided per patient. "Notable" deviations from the norms are flagged for further investigation, which is usually performed by the state Medicaid agency. The high-volume providers, physicians with a large percentage of Medicaid claims, tend to agitate the MMIS, while physicians with small benefit program practices are not likely to create any concerns unless their relatively few bills are consistently far out of line. In itself, MMIS can only provide clues and hints about possible wayward practices. The system can detect patently impossible activities, such as performing a hysterectomy on a male patient, but these are usually the result of coding errors, not fraud. Using the MMIS data, investigators develop their own methods for identifying suspicious patterns. A California agent, for instance, looks "for common surnames . . . on the computer printouts. If I see four or five members of a single family being billed for one hour individually on the same day, I'm pretty sure it isn't happening." (Of course, if family members have different surnames, this particular heuristic method will not detect any abuse.)

Computer screening has had its successes, but on the whole it has proved a less valuable tool than its progenitors envisioned. A federal staff report reviewing MMIS stated that the anticipated benefits had not been achieved and warned of "very real problems in the system."[9] The report criticized the states for failing to use MMIS on all their billings in order to develop complete profiles of providers and patients. The report also faulted the Department of Health and Human Services for certifying MMIS programs based solely on documents presented by the system's developers, rather than tests to see if the programs performed as claimed.

Once a state's MMIS program is certified, the federal government pays for 75 percent of the cost of its operation. In our survey of fifteen state MFCUs, three respondents indicated that their MMIS was of "very much" help, three judged it of "very little" help, and nine rated it as "somewhat helpful." Like all other enforcement activities, MMIS has been eviscerated by recent budget cuts. A federal official gave this example: "Take the universe of 15,000 doctors, such as in New York. They [MMIS] can still identify 450 aberrant doctors every year. It hasn't decreased. However, they can only work each year on less and less as the budget calls for less and less. But because they are working on 50 cases this year, while last year they were working on 100, doesn't mean that there are 50 less aberrant doctors out there."

Once a case is downgraded to an abuse, there is virtually no chance of a criminal prosecution. If resources allow, these cases are usually handled internally by the intermediary. The most severe sanctions that can befall the cheating physicians will be full or partial repayments of their ill-gotten funds.

Limited resources also compel investigators to decide which cases will be pursued as fraud cases and which will be downgraded to abuse cases. To prove a case of Medicaid fraud requires a finding of specific intent. Under the *Code of Federal Regulations*, Medicaid fraud is "An intentional deception or misrepresentation made by a person with the knowledge that the deception could result in some unauthorized benefit to himself or some other person. It includes any act that includes fraud under applicable federal or state law" (42 C.F.R. 1002.2). In contrast, Medicaid abuse does not require a finding of specific intent. Rather, it includes "provider practices that are inconsistent with sound fiscal, business or medical practices, and result in unnecessary cost to the Medicaid program, or reimbursement for services that are not medically necessary or that fail to meet professionally recognized standards for health care." It also includes recipient practices that result in unnecessary cost to the Medicaid program (42 C.F.R. 1001.2).

Tight budgets are not the only reason that cases of possible fraud, with its tougher sanctions, are treated as instances of abuse. Under the influence of prosecutors, who are reluctant to go forward with any but the most airtight cases, almost all investigators believe that fraud must involve "something willful." One agent offered the following rule-of-thumb distinction between fraud and abuse in the medical benefit programs:

[Fraud means] there is some intent to defraud the government and there is no question but that it's willful. . . . Abuse, on the other hand, is just basically giving people more than they need in terms of medical service—excessive treatment, treatment that is not necessary, billing for more services than are needed—anything that is above and beyond what the diagnosis calls for, but doesn't involve a willful intent. The difference between fraud and abuse, as far as I'm concerned, is in the case of fraud, services aren't rendered. In abuse cases, the services are rendered, but there is more given than is necessary based on the diagnosis.

This operating definition tells a good deal about the power that is accorded physicians to write their own fiscal ticket. It underlies the deeply cynical remark of one investigator, that fee-for-service medical benefit programs are for physicians no less than "a license to print money." To justify an array of treatments, a physician need only set forth a diagnosis that is not wildly discordant with the symptoms presented by the patient. The diagnosis will never be questioned unless a doctor's diagnosis profile appears strikingly dissimilar to those of colleagues who seemingly treat a similar clientele. If all doctors in the comparison cohort, however, are "overdiagnosing," all fall within the norms and become beyond reproach. Indeed, even if a handful are overdiagnosing, their activities can sufficiently distort what should be the norm. And even when investigators do identify a practitioner who far exceeds the norm, proving overutilization can pose almost hopeless investigative hurdles. One high-ranking official traced just such a case for us:

An internist . . . will see a patient with a certain condition six times, and I'll identify a guy who sees a patient with that condition twenty times. And now I think that somebody should tell us that this guy has seen him fourteen times too often and we should get our money back. When we put this before a medical review group, they say, "Hey, how bad is this?" Or they'll say: "Oh well, you know, it's malpractice time, and I can understand why he might have ordered unnecessary tests."

The agent's final comment reflects the belief that sharply increased outlays for malpractice insurance have affected the way physicians treat patients. There is concern that physicians practice "defensive medicine"—ordering extra diagnostic tests and performing tangential procedures, or even refusing to treat some patients for fear of litigation,[10] and refraining from performing procedures that they feel pose too much legal risk if a positive result is not obtained.[11] In 1984, in response to an AMA survey of 1,240 members, 40 percent reported they ordered additional tests to avoid lawsuits; 27 percent said they prescribed additional treatments for the same reason. More than one-third of the doctors said they spent more time with patients, 57 percent kept better patient records, 44 percent referred tough cases to other doctors, a little more than one-third no longer accepted certain kinds of cases, and 31 percent had raised their fees to recover escalated liability expenses. [12] The AMA estimated the additional cost of these tests and treatments at $15 billion to $40 billion in 1983—about 4 to 10 percent of the total yearly American health bill. [13]

Medicaid, however, pays only for "medically necessary" services, not for defensive medicine, even if the patient wants it. A high-ranking Medicaid official explained:

Ninety-nine times out of a hundred a skull X ray has very little diagnostic value to a head injury. Okay, consider a bump. You get hit in the head with a baseball bat or whatever. The doctor takes an external look at it. He could be 99 percent confident that there is no fracture serious enough to warrant a skull X ray. Great, I know that. And I have sat across the table from a doctor, and I have said to the doctor, "Doc, I want $35,000 back from you because every one of your patients that has a bump on the head you give a series of skull X rays. We both know it's medically unnecessary." My kid gets a bump on the head and I take him to the emergency room and the doctor says, "We don't really need skull X rays," and I say, "Yes we do."

This last example illustrates a point that participating physicians find particularly irksome: Services defined as precautionary treatment for the middle class are labeled overutilization and Medicaid abuse when offered to the poor. Such battles over what constitutes medically necessary services are daily occurrences in the profession's losing war with the government over who defines acceptable standards of health care. The debate also structures enforcement priorities.

Given these almost insurmountable difficulties in proving fraudulent intent on the part of a physician, enforcement officials presented with cases bordering on fraud, those in the gray area, rarely elect to pursue them. Instead, those cases are treated as instances of abuse. An administrator summarizes the situation: "One basic rule is that we should take actions only to the extent that they are actions we can defend. We've had enough experience with attorneys, hearings, and the courts, so that we've become very sensitive about the need to document the reasons for our actions to make sure they hold up."

INVESTIGATION OF
MEDICAID FRAUD

Investigators dealing with physician fraud often find themselves in an uncomfortable, awkward position in that their job requires them to confront members of a higher-status profession with allegations of misconduct. The encounters can become quite testy, when physicians are put on the defensive and have to respond to inquiries that might be incriminating and can easily be interpreted as insulting.

Our interviews indicated that experienced investigators tend to develop an occupationally useful disparagement for members of the medical profession in general. They act scrupulously polite to the doctors they investigate and then take a certain pleasure, common to law enforcers, in coldly observing the gyrations—the lies and excuses—of their prey. Some physicians attempt to face the investigators down, often with bluster. But what the doctors often fail to appreciate is that experienced investigators are familiar with the scenario, have heard all the excuses, recriminations, and lies before, though for the physician the interview is a novel experience. Some physicians appreciate or quickly learn that responsive courtesy and, if called for, sincere repentance are much more effective than aggressive combativeness.

A particularly acute problem, especially for investigators new to the job, is their lack of medical expertise. Doctors, of course, have spent a great deal of time acquiring specialized knowledge, jargon, and medical lore. Investigators, laboring in unfamiliar technical territory, can be overwhelmed or outflanked by statements they are unable to challenge. The head of fraud detection for one of the intermediaries commented wryly that the person most likely to be successful in investigating medical fraud is "a registered nurse who also is a certified public accountant and who has spent four years with the FBI." In reality, though, many investigators are former law enforcement personnel who never made it to nursing school or accounting classes.

When the investigator begins discussing the reason for his or her visit, physicians commonly deflect personal culpability by blaming their office staff. "I didn't know what my billing clerk was doing. We'll change it right away." If the violations have not been awful and if the doctor's repentance seems sincere, such a response may placate an investigator and end the inquiry. Like most regulatory agents, Medicaid investigators must continuously make compromises between a strict, tough enforcement stance and the pragmatic resolution of immediate problems.[14] General deterrence—keeping others in line by making an example of a miscreant—is not a high enforcement priority, except in cases that seem likely to command a lot of media attention. Besides, agents—and particularly their superiors—do not like to antagonize unnecessarily such prominent and potentially powerful citizens as physicians and their cohort of professional and community supporters. Exculpatory responses that are regarded as "forthcoming" and "cooperative" are likely to prompt the relabeling of offenses as "business errors," with no further action.

Because physicians are not accustomed to, or notably tolerant of, laypeople's asking for details about their work, investigators stress the importance of handling physicians with particular tact and delicacy. Asked how she goes about talking to a hostile doctor, an investigator outlined the following approach:

We would try to maintain . . . wouldn't get upset or get angry. We would let them call us all kinds of things which they come up with a lot of times. We would listen to them talk all about the bureaucracy and the terrible Medi-Cal patients that never show up for appointments, and you just let them go ahead and rave and rant and you tell them—you would never tell them that they didn't do something. You would say you billed for an injection, but we can't find the documentation for it. We are not saying that you didn't do it, but you didn't document it. We can't substantiate the code you billed. We would do it that way. And they might come back with: "I don't like to write and I am not going to."

Attempting to convey the necessity for accurate records is far more effective than lecturing about how doctors who draw money from a government program are obligated to conform to its requirements. Any approach that smacks of authoritarianism—"You'll do it because we say so"—is not considered prudent with doctors, who might well complain to an investigator's superiors or to medical authorities about high-handed zealousness. Instead, calm reason is the order of the day:

We would point out that if they are going to take Medi-Cal patients, they have to document the services. Medi-Cal is concerned with continuing care. If you walk out and get hit by a car, the doctor who . . . takes up your practice has to take care of that patient based on what you wrote. And if he doesn't know that you have done every conceivable lab test, he is going to do them all over again. But usually they don't want to write. Doctors think they are going to live forever, and are going to have those patients the rest of their lives.

It is noteworthy that this investigator attributes most cases of inadequate documentation to a combination of laziness (or an unwillingness to do work that offers no cash benefit) and a feeling of immortality. It seems a bit counterintuitive that doctors are concerned about malpractice suits but fail to take the crucial step of keeping the scrupulous records they would need to defend themselves. But if it is true that inertia rather than dishonesty lies at the heart of most inadequate billing practices, then investigators who come upon sloppy records are faced with the difficult task of differentiating physicians who cheat from lazy but honest doctors.

Most physicians, given the tactics employed by the California investigator we have been quoting, would "start documenting better, at least for a while." And the case would be put aside. But the attitude of the person under suspicion plays a significant role in the investigator's reaction. An observation about police work on the streets offers a good analogy: "In the aggregate of cases the police are more likely to arrest a misdemeanor suspect who is disrespectful to them than a felony suspect who is civil. . . . the police enforce their authority more severely than they enforce the law."[15] Similarly, physicians who indulge in truculence or hostility almost invariably generate tougher enforcement responses.

Assessments of the reliability of patients who can testify as witnesses may also play a critical role in determining whether an investigation of a physician will move forward or be dropped. Investigators commonly take one of two positions on this matter; though contradictory, both undoubtedly have elements of truth. One view is that many Medicaid patients are likely to make poor witnesses. "If you're talking about psychiatry-type cases," one investigator noted, "most of your patients are going to be borderline competent anyway. If they need psychiatric treatment, there's something wrong with them anyway. I maybe shouldn't say that, but they're not the best witnesses." Elderly patients, another investigator observed, "are a little forgetful, like I am." Occasionally, what at first seems to be fraud will prove to be a case of faulty memory. Another investigator discussed in some detail the special difficulties of interviewing patients:

Talk about agents and investigators going out and interviewing a beneficiary . . . this is not the highlight of an investigator's career. Maybe you're the only guy who's come to see her this month. And then there's the problem of getting them to remember. Did you get an injection or did you not get an injection? Did the doctor see you on a given day or did he not? It can be a very frustrating type of thing, especially if you've got a doctor who is going to a nursing home and walking through the rooms and taking the names of patients. Dealing with nursing home patients is even worse because most of them will not make good witnesses.

There is irony here: Physicians who pick particularly weak and infirm people to victimize improve their chances of getting away with it.

Other investigators, however, tell stories showing that some Medicaid patients prove to be better witnesses than anyone might have thought. "Patients, believe it or not," says a New York investigator, "have pretty good memories about when they went to the doctor and when they didn't." They write their appointments on a calendar, and some have to summon a taxicab in order to get to the doctor, so there may be a formal record of the occasion. In inactive lives, a trip to the doctor can be memorable, the details remaining firmly implanted in the patient's memory. Another investigator thought that cheating physicians tended to be careless because they underestimated the intelligence of their Medicaid patients: "They think that welfare patients are stupid, and I think that's their biggest mistake because there are a lot of bright people on public assistance and we go out and interview those people."

MFCUs: UNDERCOVER
OPERATIONS AND STINGS

One step in our research on the investigation of Medicaid fraud cases was to survey MFCUs throughout the United States. We sent questionnaires to the thirty existing programs, but only nineteen supplied information, despite an accompanying letter of support from the president of the national MFCU association and our emphasis in the cover letter that our work was funded by the U.S. Department of Justice. We also assured respondents of anonymity.

The explanation most often given by MFCU directors for not responding to our survey was that their units had been burned by a congressional staff report based on their answers to a federal inquiry. The essence of that report is captured by its subtitle, which maintained that there was a "failure in state enforcement."[16] The state MFCUs were thus not inclined to cooperate with us. Nonetheless, with almost two-thirds of the units responding and through telephone queries to other units, we obtained a general portrait of their work and concerns.

Although the units differ notably in size, each MFCU employs attorneys, auditors, investigators, and support staff. Such staffing mixes are required to qualify for federal funds, and they are based on the early experience of New York's special Medicaid fraud unit, which predated the federal authorization of the MFCUs. Typically, investigators and auditors outnumber other jobholders in the MFCUs. Of the nineteen units responding to our survey, eleven had more auditors than attorneys, three had the opposite distribution, and five had equal numbers of each.

The MFCUs also differ in their investigative powers and law enforcement status. In almost half the states with MFCUs (eighteen of thirty-eight), fraud investigators are not sworn peace officers and therefore cannot arrest suspected wrongdoers or directly secure subpoenas. Nor can they carry a weapon or routinely use electronic wiretapping or body bugs. These restrictions were said to undermine the morale of MFCU personnel and hinder their efficient resolution of cases. Obtaining information about a suspect becomes especially painstaking and frustrating when an MFCU does not have its own prosecutor and must go before a grand jury each time it wishes to secure a subpoena. Eliciting the cooperation of prosecuting attorneys in the district attorney's office can also be troublesome, since few Medicaid fraud cases produce headlines that will advance a young prosecutor's career. Nor is prosecuting a physician whose livelihood and liberty are at stake a cakewalk. Some physicians fight back savagely and have the resources to mount formidable legal defenses.

The head of an MFCU outlined for us some of the juridical considerations that arise in cases of physician fraud:

To do a white-collar crime takes a lot of teamwork. Your grand juries have to be available, your subpoenas have to be timely. . . . These things are very, very important. They can't be piecemeal. You cannot go out and conduct a good white-collar crime investigation by just utilizing the services of the so-called "good investigator and auditor." It won't work because someplace along the line, you're going to be stiffed. Then you have to go to a district attorney or a federal prosecutor who really is not trained, nor does he have the patience to do a white-collar crime investigation. White-collar crime calls for a lot of patience, and most of the young attorneys want to go into the court with John Dillinger by the nape of the neck, and it just doesn't work that way.

To obtain sufficient evidence to sustain a charge of Medicaid fraud, undercover operations are often essential. Seventeen of the nineteen responding MFCUs reported no trouble securing Medicaid cards for undercover work ("shopping" in the investigators' lingo) directly from the state Medicaid agency. At the time, one state required that "reasonable suspicion" be shown by affidavit before a magistrate would issue a card—but this policy has since been changed, and now the director of the state Department of Health can issue Medicaid cards to undercover police officers. The first pair of agents who applied for cards in order to "shop" a physician, however, received cards numbered 001 and 002—a gaffe they wryly regarded as illustrating both the stupidity of the state administrative agency and its indifference to effective monitoring.

Despite their potential for securing valuable evidence, shopping forays were used sparingly by the MFCUs. Nine of the nineteen MFCUs indicated they had not used shopping to investigate a physician within the past year; seven units reported three or fewer shopping investigations in the same period. A major concern, mentioned by nine of the respondents, was that shopping expeditions could be construed by the court as entrapment.

Practical limitations on shopping forays were also cited. To investigate providers who see patients only through referrals, undercover agents would first have to be examined by a general practitioner or internist. In small rural and suburban communities, the sudden appearance of an outsider-patient would provoke suspicion. Cost and time constraints also inhibit the use of shopping. Proving criminal intent beyond a reasonable doubt can require multiple transactions by several operatives, with backup personnel on or near the scene.

Concern with the safety and health of the undercover agents also figured prominently among the concerns of the MFCUs. One referred to the possible risk of hepatitis from contaminated needles and "exposure to unhealthy persons and surroundings." Another noted the "risks of [the] investigator investigating MDs who examine the investigator to prescribe medicine." Life-threatening situations are quite rare, but not unheard of. One investigator reported the following unnerving experience: "We went into the doctor's office, and he sat at his desk. . . . When I glanced over at him, he had a gun sitting in his lap, pointing at [another investigator]." In another case, a California physician was charged with solicitation for murder after he allegedly paid $75,000 to a former patient to have an MFCU investigator and a witness against him in a Medicaid fraud case murdered to prevent them from testifying. The state Board of Medical Quality Assurance declared the doctor was suffering from "severe paranoid schizophrenia," though the prosecuting attorney adopted a more prosaic view, noting that the physician, by filing slander suits against witnesses and prosecutors, had successfully delayed the criminal proceeding against him. "[He] knows what he is doing and manipulates the system," the prosecutor insisted.[17]

About half the respondents cited the issue of agents' credibility as patients. If a doctor is to believe that an agent is a legitimate patient, the agent must fit in with the doctor's speciality and clientele. Scrutinizing the activities of a geriatric specialist or a pediatrician, or investigating a doctor whose practice focuses on a single ethnic group, cannot be done by just any undercover agent.

This requirement proved to be a significant stumbling block in a controversial Medicaid fraud case that arose in a Westminster community (nicknamed "Little Saigon") in Southern California. There were no Asian investigators on the enforcement staff; ultimately, an informant with less than an immaculate background was recruited to observe sales of Medicaid stickers by program beneficiaries to "drivers" employed by physicians. Doctors then submitted the stickers for reimbursement for medical services they had not performed. The use of such drivers reflected a practice in provincial Vietnamese villages, by which some doctors paid pedicab drivers or "bicycle boys" to solicit patients and drive them to their clinics. The Westminster drivers were paid $4 to $7 for each Medi-Cal case they secured. The physicians simply peeled off stickers and billed Medi-Cal from $12 to $56 for each "examination." They then would add blood, urine, and other tests. A sudden increase in the number of physicians in the area was said to have led to vicious competition.[18] At the end of the investigation, ten of the fifty Vietnamese doctors practicing in Westminster were arrested in a media circus attended by the state attorney general and Mike Wallace of "60 Minutes" (though the filmed material was never televised).

This episode was notably different from the usual Medi-Cal prosecution. Tip-offs about the alleged fraud came from "several unrelated letters" written by members of the community. The flamboyant arrest procedure, with suspects handcuffed to chairs in the jail parking lot while the photographers clicked away, differed dramatically from any previous apprehension of physicians. Racism may well have been an issue; at the least, the raid indicated insensitivity to the meaning of loss of face in Asian culture. The ruses enforcement agents allegedly employed to gather evidence elicited protests from such groups as the Federation of Vietnamese Catholics on the West Coast, which noted, "sources state that, as a rule they [the investigators] used strong and menacing words such as the immediate suspension of government assistance or arrest by police, and tried to frighten Vietnamese refugees into admission of their involvement in the sale of Medi-Cal [coupons]. In some cases, investigators began their inquiries by menacingly throwing handcuffs on the table of their hosts."[19]

Most of those arrested pled guilty to a variety of offenses and were sentenced to probation and restitution. Five physicians received jail or prison terms. In the only case that went to trial, however, a doctor and an alleged driver were acquitted—two years after the arrests. Milton Grimes, the attorney for the acquitted defendants, insisted that the earlier guilty pleas had come because the authorities had "stampeded" the doctors. He argued and persuaded the jury that his clients had been entrapped. The jury foreman later noted, "There was not one witness that had a bad thing to say about [the defendant doctor], whether by reputation, or that he was involved in any way, shape, or form" in the illegal purchase of Medi-Cal coupons. During the trial, the undercover agent, himself a former driver, testified that he believed that "entrapment" could be defined as "using force to get someone to do what you want, using a gun or knife." "Did you employ a gun or a knife?" asked Grimes. The agent laughingly dismissed such a preposterous idea, but he failed to appreciate that he had misinterpreted the law on entrapment, which does not require the physical coercion he presumed it did. [20]

To avoid the difficulties of finding agents who could be credible patients, several MFCUs suggested that shopping of doctors for fraud ought to be carried out by enlisting volunteers among the physician's actual patients. Two units expressed an interest in mounting "sting" operations—such as the FBI's Abscam foray against congressmen—in which physicians strongly suspected of cheating would be tempted—but not entrapped—by contrived situations to commit violations. [21] Another MFCU head favored using electronic eavesdropping devices in undercover operations. Juries were said to have been "spoiled" by Abscam and to have turned skeptical about evidence that failed to include a videotape of the charged behavior. The use of such tactics against Medicaid fraud is illustrated in a case description:

We had a fellow. He opened a nursing home. He was in serious trouble, and we figured if he would cooperate with law enforcement, maybe we could suggest to the judge who was going to sentence him that he would consider his cooperation. He thought that was a good idea and asked, "What can I do for you?" We said if we put a microphone in your home, will you invite all the various providers—cleaning people, meat guys. Every single one offered him a kickback—25 percent to 40 percent.

Two MFCUs pointed out that speed was a key factor in investigating cases, particularly when witnesses' memories were important for effective prosecution. Undercover work, they maintained, was too inefficient to be useful:

Our unit now uses a method of intercepting claims when [they are] filed. Recipients associated with suspect claims are then interviewed as soon as possible. This eliminates witness memory problems. It is more efficient than undercover operations because a greater number of instances are uncovered in a shorter period of time, and one investigator produces a greater number of provable instances than if he shopped as an undercover operative.

Another MFCU advocated more extensive use of polygraph tests; one unit thought a Medicaid hotline for reporting suspected providers was a useful enforcement aid. The installation of such a toll-free state hotline generated twelve hundred to fifteen hundred calls a month and had become a chief source of prosecutor information. One-third of the calls were reported to have good potential.

Asked to rate various items that might affect the cases they pursue, the MFCUs ranked as "always important" evidence considerations (14 units), patient's welfare (12 units), and the dollar amount of the suspected fraud (10 units). Rated as "not important" by all but one of the units was the power of the doctor involved in the case. In many respects, the ratings reflect the prosecutors' priorities, because investigators almost invariably focus on only those cases they believe will appeal to prosecutors. An agent described how his office ascertained whether they and the prosecutors were on the same wavelength:

Very early on in the investigation, before we expend a lot of investigative resources, we'll go directly to the prosecutor and make a presentation. . . . We'll set forth the allegations and facts as developed preliminarily and then ask the prosecutor, "If we substantiate these allegations, given the dollar amounts, the proofs, and so forth, will you prosecute this case?" So we are right up front in our system of priorities whether or not to make a commitment of our resources or end it right there.

An agent usually has to sell the prosecutor on the case. In effect, allegations of provider fraud must compete with other federal or state offenses for the attention of the district or U.S. attorney. An investigator commenting on federal prosecutors noted, "Their priorities are bank robberies, drugs, immigration, and terrorists. The work load of the assistants is huge. Somebody goes and blows up nine airplanes, and then you come in the next day with a doctor who is [stealing] from Medicare or Medicaid. Where are the priorities? They will be more concerned with violent crimes."

Judging the suitability of a case for prosecution involves balancing considerations that bear upon both the heinousness of the behavior and the cost-benefit ratio in terms of other demands on the prosecuting office's time and resources. A federal investigator, talking about Medicare, supplies an analysis that is equally appropriate for Medicaid:

The first thing they always looked at is money. You can't get a guy whose [fraudulent] bills are $3,000 to $4,000 a year. No matter how good the complaint is, it's probably not going to warrant federal prosecution. Then you get into other questions. How much work are we going to have to do on this case? Are you talking about a guy adding an injection where he's getting an extra $2 per claim so that you're going to have to interview a thousand or two thousand people? If that were the case, he may feel that it's better [to pursue] civil action. The fact is that there is going to be a lot of work. Just because there's going to be a lot of work shouldn't be a criterion, and it usually isn't. But there are times where you have somebody bucking for one or two dollars per claim. The amount of evidence you need to prove it beyond a reasonable doubt . . . just becomes burdensome.

The same respondent also stressed that the weight of the evidence plays an important role in the prosecutor's decisions:

If it's an open-and-shut case where this guy is obviously committing a fraud and the intent is there, and the evidence is there . . . it may not be a lot of money, but the evidence is going to outweigh it, and so they may prosecute it. Usually if you get patient abuse, that may not overwhelm the assistant [federal attorney], but a lot of times that may be the extra thing. Say the guy's taking X rays with no film in it, or he's allowing his secretary to prescribe drugs; then sometimes that will outweigh some of the other factors. It's kind of a scale. The amount of dollars is taken into effect, the amount of work, or what you're going to have to prove. On the other side is, what is the evidence going to show? Is it going to be overwhelming? Is he really fooling around with the patients' welfare?

The MFCUs suggested that certain groups of medical providers had more dishonest members than others. Those they viewed as particularly prone to cheating were doctors specializing in obstetrics and gynecology, psychiatrists, dentists, pharmacists, nursing home operators, ambulance companies, and medical supply businesses. Chiropractors were regarded as comparatively honest.

The sanctions to prevent physician fraud deemed to be "effective" or "very effective" by the MFCUs were delicensing from practice (19 responses), jail or prison terms (17), suspension from participation in benefit programs (15), media publicity (14), and professional sanctions (14). Fines, recovery of funds, and administrative sanctions were seen as of lesser value. The MFCUs viewed community service, a popular option with some judges, as a notably ineffective sanction. (This last view corresponds with that of well-regarded criminologists Marshall Clinard and Peter Yeager, whose research on corporate crime and judicial responses to it led them to recommend that community service in place of incarceration should be prohibited by law, except for very unusual circumstances.)[22]

The MFCUs try to court the media, but they have to compete with juicier cases that grab more newspaper and television attention and that offer more spectacular photo and video opportunities. One MFCU blamed the media's lack of interest in part on the unwillingness of judges to impose severe sentences—accompanied by fiery personal denouncements—that might appeal to news-gathering organizations: "We haven't had any real publicity on any of the cases that have been made in the state. There have been no real big splashes, mainly because there have been no real good convictions. We've had convictions, but they've all been very lightly sentenced and therefore no big wow in the press. . . . I think that's one of the most important things . . . the publicity you can get with a harsh sentence." Moreover, as this administrator pointed out, few cases go to trial. Guilty pleas, rather than trials, tend to be the order of the day, "simply because of the nature of the profession. They don't want too much embarrassment, and they know they'll get light sentences."

Few units suggested structural alterations in the benefit programs as a way to reduce fraud and abuse. Of those that did have a suggestion, the change most often mentioned was a switch from fee-for-service to a health maintenance organization (HMO) style of care. Then, physicians would be on salary and would presumably lack personal financial incentives to cheat. One MFCU respondent believed that HMOs would be much easier to monitor and that HMO doctors would behave creditably: "They've got a patient, and they are going to get *x* amount of dollars from that patient. Take care of his whole needs. If [a patient] doesn't get any service, we can prove that. If a doctor does that to one [patient], he's going to do it to more than one, so we can find that—no service and still billing. That's fraud . . . and I don't really have that terrible feeling about doctors as far as treatment goes. I think they see a sick person, they're going to treat him."

Other measures suggested to reduce fraud were a requirement for authorization before services could be rendered—a matter particularly irksome to doctors—and some form of patient copayment. A number of states now demand prior authorization for particular services before they will pay a physician, particularly one deemed an overutilizer. The premise of a patient copayment system is that beneficiaries will become more active consumers because they will have to pay at least a small part of the bill. Medical services, however, seem not to respond very well to traditional marketplace considerations: Consumers rarely comparison-shop for the best deal—a behavior that seriously frustrates attempts to control physicians' billing practices.

Investigators also feel hamstrung in many jurisdictions by their inability to obtain information from private insurers. They maintain that if they could obtain a complete picture of a physician's practice, putting together private and Medicaid billing patterns, they could more easily identify violations. Securing records from private insurers, however, involves questions of privacy and confidentiality and often requires a grand jury subpoena. Access to medical records brings into conflict two highly regarded American values: the government's right to determine how its funds are spent and the patient's and physicians' right to expect that medical records remain confidential. Early in the nation's history, doctor-patient privilege was not defined by statute. In 1793, for example, a doctor's testimony obtained in medical confidence was compelled in a divorce action based on adultery. The first statute making communications between doctor and patient privileged was enacted by New York in 1928. Today, two-thirds of the states have similar statutes.[23]

The courts, after balancing the government's regulatory interest against the patient's privacy interest, have often allowed disclosure of medical records. Although some courts have limited the extent of the information that can be disclosed, few have set forth explicit standards to protect medical records from unwarranted disclosure of confidential information.[24] Even when investigators have obtained permission from patients to review their records, judges have held that medical confidentiality takes precedence over government attempts to detect fraud or that the government's mission could just as well be served by using other investigative techniques.[25] Such rulings frustrate investigators, who suspect that physicians—especially psychiatrists—sometimes use the cloak of confidentiality to camouflage wrongdoing; these investigators resent physicians who offer high-minded defenses to conceal criminal behavior.

PROSECUTING MEDICAID CASES

The laws creating MFCUs, as noted, required that the units be placed in agencies that had their own prosecutorial resources. In those states where such placement is illegal, however, MFCU investigators must persuade district and federal attorneys to include medical fraud violations in their heavy caseloads. One investigator noted cynically some of the problems with initiating prosecutions: "We can't prove intent for a number of reasons. One, no one would suspect this upstanding pillar of the comunity of any fraudulent intent. He has a tremendous education, makes a great appearance. He is in that social order that is making the decisions [about] whether he is right or wrong—judges, prosecutors." The size of the community in which a case arises also affects how the prosecution is handled. The head of the Arkansas MFCU, for instance, noted that he prefers a federal prosecutor to handle his cases, in part because of greater experience and resources but also because "a small-town prosecutor, holding elective office, may be unenthusiastic about prosecuting a prominent local physician."[26]

The allegation that the class congruity between the higher functionaries in the criminal justice system and the suspected offenders protects doctors from prosecution echoes a point about white-collar crime that Edwin Sutherland made in the 1940s. In his meticulous manner, Sutherland worked his way through the kinds of relationships between the well-off that lead them to protect each other: "Persons in government are, by and large, culturally homogeneous with persons in business." Besides, "many persons in government are members of families which have other members in business." In addition, Sutherland cited close personal connections between many businessmen and government officials, and noted that many persons in government had at one time worked for a company in an executive capacity or hoped to do so in the future. Sutherland also mentioned the government's particular concern about not antagonizing business because of its power and significance as a source of funds for political campaigns. All told, he maintained, "the initial cultural homogeneity, the close personal relationships, and the power relationships protect businessmen against critical definitions by government."[27]

Indeed, although powerful people may attract disproportionate critical attention, the records of American politics are replete with stories of prosecutors being told to drop a case after somebody had gotten to their higher-ups, often political appointees.[28] But MFCU investigators do not regard upper-class solidarity as the major obstacle to securing prosecutions. Instead, they cite the fact that most prosecutors lack the expertise essential for the successful handling of medical fraud cases:

White-collar crime calls for a lot of patience. . . . We just successfully prosecuted a nursing home operator [after seven years on the case]. . . . He stiffed us. First of all he fought our subpoenas. Then he fought our grand jury authority. Then he fought this, then he fought that, then he appealed this, then he appealed that. And the judicial system we have, it's a democracy, we have to accept it, we have to live with it. But in order to catch these people and do any kind of reasonably good job, we have to go this route. There is no district attorney's office nor U.S. attorney's office—they come into office every four years or every eight years—that can handle this kind of prosecutorial situation. They don't have the patience for it. And further, there's an awful lot of different little types of techniques that a lawyer has to have with these kinds of cases. Another thing, the judges don't like these cases.

An agent in Florida offered a similar observation: "These smaller circuits, all they're doing is rapes, robberies, murders, B & Es [breaking and entering]. You can try a good murder case in probably three or four days, whereas a white-collar crime could take three or four weeks. You can walk in with a wheelbarrow full of documentary evidence. They're apprehensive about trying them. They're complex, take a lot of time, a lot of preparation." A federal official spoke to the same theme: "Most prosecutors are young people, relatively new out of school, and they break, you know, cut their teeth on gun cases and buy or bust drug cases. You're trying to build your record around the community as a good lawyer, and you go off on a two-year investigation, and people don't know you're around anymore. That's the down side of doing fraud cases."

Prosecutorial strategy typically involves selecting those charges easiest to prove, rather than placing all possible violations before the jury. "You don't list as a basis for a charge every single rotten thing the guy did because you would bore the court and jury to death." All the while, the clock is running—the statute of limitations is generally five years.

According to the investigators, prosecutors believe that judges and juries are reluctant to convict physicians, and therefore prosecutors accept only those cases of fraud that can be expected to result in a conviction or a guilty plea. It is arguable, but unlikely, that investigators themselves are hesitant or uncomfortable about pursuing the cases and cite the biases of those more powerful in the decision-making process merely to justify their own behaviors.

Overzealousness in prosecuting physicians can backfire, as is illustrated by a 1985 case in which a Honolulu optician faced a jury trial for having charged the state $7.75 each for four eyeglass nose pads he had not provided. The head of the Hawaii MFCU, under attack by the press, insisted, "A person's honesty does not depend on how much he steals, but whether he steals at all." The governor, though, said the case "bothered him." After the doctor was acquitted, the MFCU administrator was fired.[29]

Cases not accepted by prosecutors are usually referred back to the health departments or to intermediaries or carriers for civil or administrative actions. Penalties include the repayment of misappropriated funds, a requirement that all services be approved for payment in advance, and suspension from the Medicaid program (which also entails suspension from Medicare). Whatever the outcome, few members of the public will ever hear about the wrongdoing, and the deterrent effect on other providers will be minimal.

PUNISHING MEDICAID FRAUD

Considerable behavioral science literature insists that punishment of white-collar and professional offenders is apt to be notably effective in deterring recidivists and in deterring persons tempted to commit abuses.[30] Such conclusions are based on two suppositions: first, that white-collar offenders have a great deal to lose by prosecution, and so they will be much more disinclined than other offenders to take risks if they suspect they will be caught; second, that white-collar offenses are essentially rational behaviors, the product of utilitarian calculation—rather than of passion, sociopathic personality disorders, or desperation—and that white-collar criminals are thus more likely to weigh the likelihood of detection and punishment than other offenders.

There exist no means to test these propositions in regard to Medicaid fraud (or, for that matter, in regard to crime in general). For one thing, to the extent that medical criminals correctly perceive the limits to detection, enforcement, and sanctioning—the lax enforcement and weak sentences—the deterrent efficacy of punishment is reduced. In the case of physician lawbreaking in the Medicaid program, those who view the system itself as illegitimate are apt to be less influenced by the threat of legal sanctions. Overall, the efficacy of deterrence depends heavily on the ability of the law enforcement apparatus to apply sanctions effectively to violators—a condition highly questionable in the case of both common and white-collar crime.[31]

An investigative supervisor in New York maintains that "doctors' earnings go down when they realize they're being investigated." But even if one grants that this observation is accurate, one cannot be sure that being under investigation prompts physicians to recommit themselves to law-abiding behavior, or merely to a temporary prudence until the investigation is concluded.

Most investigators deplore the failure of the courts to impose jail or prison sentences on convicted Medicaid malefactors, and they believe that the professional medical associations are notoriously indulgent of members against whom Medicaid fraud has been proven. Physician-controlled medical boards rarely suspend the right to practice and commonly regard the crimes as merely a business matter, not as a reflection on professional competence. An investigator noted:

You never can get any doctor delicensed for being a thief. They won't take his license away because that really has nothing to do with his expertise. If he did something wrong to the patient, the fixing of the patient, that is something else altogether. As far as being a thief, overbilling, double-billing, services not rendered, forget it. It never really gets to the heart of kicking him out. They can kick him out of Medicaid, but who the hell cares about Medicaid. The guy's still making bucks.

A California doctor working with a licensing agency summarized the situation from his vantage point: "Unless a guy really, you know, has been blatant, blatant about his fraud, he usually doesn't lose his license. What we usually do is to put him on probation, restitution to the Department of Health. . . . One of the most important terms in probation is an imposition of community free medical care and in, you know, some needed area, for a number of years, maybe for six to eight hours a week." Even this seemingly straightforward resolution has not been without sardonic twists. Another official told us that clinics had billed Medi-Cal for services provided by physicians who had been sentenced to offer free care at such sites.

Only rarely do judges sentence doctors convicted of Medicaid fraud to prison terms. In part, the incongruity of regarding doctors as "real" criminals appears to protect them from incarceration. In other instances, a convicted physician is seen as providing a vital service that cannot readily be replaced, especially in underserviced communities. A federal official tells about the disposition of the case of a doctor who had been convicted in three separate cases:

There was a case in Philadelphia [of a doctor] who got nailed for the third time. The first time it was for IRS fraud. The second time it was Medicaid, and then he came up a third time on Medicare. When the doctor showed up to be sentenced, he brought in his Medicare population who were going to be disadvantaged by his being gone. So the judge came up with a fairly creative sentence. He gave him weekends. The guy practiced during the week, and on weekends, we assume he went to jail.

The common tactic of excluding convicted doctors for a period of time—usually a few years—from further participation in Medicaid and Medicare seems to be a relatively benign consequence, though for doctors dependent on the benefit programs for most of their livelihood, the deprivations are hurtful—until they locate other sources of income.

The original Medicaid legislation provided only for recovery of over-payments, not for suspension. In 1977, however, suspension was made automatic if a physician was convicted in a federal, state, or local court for defrauding the system (Public Law 95-142). A legal notice of suspension must be published in a local newspaper (and in a Spanish-language newspaper where appropriate) after a letter of notification is sent to the provider. The first claim received from a beneficiary who goes to a suspended doctor will be paid, but a notice is sent to the beneficiary pointing out that no further claim involving that provider will be honored.

An official's summary of a suspension case indicates that even a suspension can be undone:

We have a provider in Minnesota who was convicted. . . . They were faking insurance claims with private insurance companies, faking workmen's comp, and billing Medicaid for services that weren't rendered. . . . He went to jail for two months and then decided he would suddenly become a humanitarian, so he moved to West Virginia to work in a camp for asthmatic underprivileged children, and suddenly became an expert in that field, and set himself up as being indispensable to the underprivileged and to a medically underrepresented community.

His hearing [to remove the suspension] was held in a different region, and they thought he was a real nice guy, and the law judge lowered our ten-year suspension to a two-year period and then decided that if we had done everything as quickly as he thought we could have, the suspension would have been put into effect two years ago. So he didn't say make it retroactive, but he basically made it retroactive. And the guy got away with a sixty-eight- or sixty-two-day suspension.

Most enforcement personnel strongly favor tough penalties and in-carceration for doctors who engage in fraud, but they grant that such outcomes are improbable. Instead, enforcement has begun to concen-trate heavily on recovering illegally gained monies and imposing fines. In 1981, section 2105 of Public Law 95-35 authorized fines for fraud against government health care programs.[32] Under this statute the secretary of HHS can impose a penalty of up to $2,000 for each fraudulent medical claim and can impose an assessment of up to twice the amount of the fraudulent portion of the claim in lieu of damages.

One advantage of the administratively handled civil penalty, which does not preclude criminal prosecution, is that civil cases have a lower standard of proof—"preponderance of evidence" is the criterion—com-pared to the criminal code, which requires the prosecution to prove wrongdoing "beyond a reasonable doubt." Civil libertarians, however, are dissatisfied by the distinction between a civil fine and a criminal fine. In *Trop v. Dulles*, a deportation case, Chief Justice Earl Warren wrote, "a statute that prescribes the consequence that will befall one who fails to abide by these regulatory provisions is a penal law." Even a clear legislative classification of a statute as nonpenal, Warren wrote, would not alter the fundamental nature of a plainly penal statute. Nonetheless, in *Chapman v. U.S.* the Tenth Circuit Court of Appeals ruled that under the Medicaid law, a civil fine is not a criminal penalty.[33]

Investigators also find the civil penalty provisions advantageous be-cause criminal court judges, whom the investigators regard as indul-gent, are not involved. The fraud penalties handed down by judges who are used to sentencing violent criminals tend to be too light, complained one former MFCU director:

A classic case. We did a complete, comprehensive audit on a lab operator which established without any question $300,000 of bilking the state. . . . We went in and got another one of those gutless judges who said: "Oh, he's a professional man; he's suffered enough having to go through the criminal process. And therefore even though he pleaded guilty, I am going to require him to pay only half of the restitution." So we get $160,000 from this guy, and we were outraged. The rest is profit. Who wouldn't go into crime?

Such concern about the white-collar defendant having "suffered enough" is not unusual. Judges recognize that damage to a physician's reputation is a form of punishment in itself. As one Medicaid official noted, "You put [a doctor's] name on the front page of the paper as a thief, you've destroyed him." In contrast, the destruction of a street offender's life, livelihood, and family is somehow viewed more cavalierly, as though a defendant who had little to begin with has nothing much to lose from a criminal conviction. In this peculiar bit of folk wisdom, falls from high places are the stuff of tragedy, but the tumbles of those who had not climbed so high are assumed to be less painful—the latter are supposed to suffer less because they are accustomed to having so little. Nonetheless, judges typically refer to the loss of standing already experienced by a white-collar offender as a basis for a light sentence.

Unlike typical street offenders who have scant income or assets, however, well-heeled physicians are worth pursuing civilly and worth assessing costs against. In California, civil fines carry 25 percent interest, and the adjudicated provider must also pay the expenses of the audit that formed the basis of the case. In Florida, judges are authorized to levy investigative costs against a provider. An official noted that "we've used [this penalty] as a plea-negotiating line, and it's been very effective that way." Florida officials estimate that more than a quarter of a million dollars in investigative costs were recovered by this means between 1984 and 1988. A New Jersey court ruled that such costs may include the expense of investigatory work as well as the preparation of administrative and appellate hearings. New York mandates that fraudulent activities in regard to medical benefit programs may be punished by the imposition of treble damages. Because a restitution order does not debar a victim from suing, the state can also move against an offender in court, but this tactic is generally used only as a last resort, following deep dissatisfaction with an administrative disposition.

TACTICS OF TIGHTROPE
ENFORCEMENT

All law enforcement efforts in the United States are constrained by public opinion as well as legal curbs on government activity. For example, a notably efficient method for detecting income tax fraud—by employing many thousands more investigators—probably would so infuriate the public that an administration proposing such a measure would find itself in political difficulty. Similarly, airport security can go only so far in hindering the pace of air traffic, and campaigns against theft can employ only a limited repertoire of techniques without running up against constitutional and political issues.[34]

In addition, law enforcement in the Medicaid fraud arena has to contend with the attitudes of care providers. As discussed in chapter 2, "the widespread fear, ground in the bitter, hostile propaganda of the AMA, that physicians would refuse to provide services under a national health program" motivated Congress to grant innumerable concessions to practitioners in the drafting of the Medicaid and Medicare bills.[35] Continuing concern about withdrawal from the programs is a major point of tension in current enforcement efforts. Program administrators continually warn investigators, as one of them told us, "If you put doctors in jail, pretty soon none of the doctors will be in Medicaid." Another official noted, "One thing we do not want to do is to dry up the pool of physicians . . . among whom the drop in the assignment rate is alarmingly high." Fearful of alienating physicians, the government practices a form of "tightrope enforcement." Investigators must attempt to prove criminal behavior without offending the profession as a whole or too many members of it.

Are such fears reasonable? The statistical picture is mixed. On one hand, only 6 percent of physicians care for one-third of the nation's Medicaid patients. In the early 1980s, one-quarter of all primary-care physicians refused to accept Medicaid patients, largely because of the low reimbursement rates.[36] A comprehensive inquiry in Pennsylvania in 1987 found that during a fifteen-month period, less than one-half of the state's 28,000 doctors had treated a Medicaid patient in their office. Slightly more than 2,000 physicians treated an average of at least one such patient a day. Interestingly, in 1986 Pennsylvania enacted a law allowing state officials to consider as an element of licensing decisions a physician's willingness to accept Medicaid patients.[37]

Despite these data from Pennsylvania, Medicaid has now become so intricately involved in medical practice that fears of massive physician withdrawal seem to be meaningless bluffs. In California, for instance, 15 percent of practicing physicians derive more than a quarter of their income from Medi-Cal patients.[38] With competition for patients becoming even more intense in some urban areas because of an alleged surplus of doctors, it hardly appears reasonable to suspect droves of doctors will abandon Medicaid merely because of more intense efforts to combat fraud. Administrative red tape and reimbursement schedules are much more likely to be of concern to Medicaid physicians.

CONCLUSION

The recent history of medical fraud and abuse adds to the argument that white-collar offenders benefit notably from a policy of benign neglect, largely traceable to their ability to impose their own definitions of acceptable professional conduct upon those who might be in a position to bring about tougher regulation. To date, the medical profession has been particularly adept at insulating its members from effective criminal action for fraudulent behavior. In part because of the profession's status and power, laws and rules cannot be stringently enforced with the resources allocated for the job—and there is no public clamor to increase those resources. Only a change in the programs' structure is likely to reduce the level of fraud significantly.

Chapter Four

What the Doctors Did

Organized medicine claims that it can police itself, but the record of Medicaid fraud and abuse indicates that the profession is unable to ferret out and punish errant doctors. If doctors who cheat are, as the profession's elite argue, only "the few rotten apples" in an otherwise pristine barrel, one would expect the medical associations to have an efficient control mechanism to spot and remove them quickly. However, few errant doctors are brought to enforcement's attention through professional channels. Rather, most physician offenses are uncovered by government fraud-control activities or are reported by former employees or current patients. And most of these offenses are committed by physicians in private practice, illustrating that Medicaid abuse is not exclusively the domain of doctors at work in inner-city Medicaid mills.

In this chapter we use case file material to tell the story of physicians' criminality. We also discuss the demographics of physicians sanctioned for violations of the Medicaid laws. We have removed all references to physicians' names. Our cases are drawn primarily from California and New York, because these two states have the largest number of violators and because their enforcement agents were cooperative in granting us access to files. Many states, as well as the Inspector General's Office at the Department of Health and Human Services, were unwilling to allow us access, most often because the files included the names of beneficiaries and the cost of removing the names was said to be prohibitive. On occasion, we have supplemented our case file material with professional or government reports or other reports that received attention in the press.

The apprehended doctors come from many specialties, and the details of their crimes are often shaped by their medical specialties. Some specialties seem to invite more misbehavior and easier apprehension; others may provide less room for abuse or may effectively shield malefactors from detection.

Like most statistics on lawbreakers, these cases tell us at least as much about enforcement patterns and priorities as about the actual distribution of crimes. Enforcement resources tend to be allocated to cases in which the dollar amounts are high, the aberrancies identified by computer checks are striking, the intent to commit fraud is reasonably clear, and the case seems relatively simple to prosecute successfully—all matters that recommend action to a prosecutor who has great discretion about which cases to accept. Cases involving unnecessary tests and procedures, for instance, receive much less attention than those in which bills are submitted for services never rendered, because the former are apt to involve a labyrinthine "paper chase" in which intent is extremely difficult to establish. How careful a physician is in defrauding Medicaid also influences the probability of discovery. The sloppiest and least clever crooks are most likely to be snared. Such matters influence the aggregate characteristics of physician violators who comprise the "official record" of known Medicaid fraud cases.

DEMOGRAPHICS

To obtain a general picture of physician violators and their offenses during the early years of enforcement, we obtained lists of providers suspended from participation in Medicare or Medicaid between 1977 and 1982. Federal law now requires that any physician or other health care professional convicted of a crime related to participation in Medicaid, Medicare, or other social service programs be suspended from participation in Medicare. Medicare suspension usually prompts Medicaid suspension, although a state can elect to continue to pay a provider who has been suspended from the federal program.

Of the 358 medical providers suspended during the period in question, 147 were physicians. Of the 138 physicians for whom we were able to obtain background information, 50 (36 percent) were graduates of overseas medical schools. Six of the forty-three schools mentioned had more than one graduate among the sanctioned doctors. Three physicians had graduated from the University of Havana, and two came from each of the following schools: Central University of Manila; Far Eastern Institute of Medicine, Manila; University of Innsbruck; University of Bologna; and the Medical University of Nuevo León in Mexico.

Among the eighty-eight domestically trained doctors, six had trained at Meharry Medical College, followed by the University of California, Irvine (five); Loma Linda in California (four); and the University of Louisville (three). Among the fifteen other schools that logged two graduates on the government list were such preeminent institutions as Johns Hopkins, the University of Wisconsin, UCLA, Tulane, New York University, and Columbia.

The disproportionate number of foreign graduates among the violators is striking. They constituted approximately 25 percent of doctors at work in the United States and 31 percent of the known violators. Also unexpected was the number of sanctioned doctors from Meharry Medical College, whose student body is predominantly black; black doctors made up only about 3 percent of the 400,000 physicians practicing in the United States at the time of our research. These results seem to reflect the heavier concentrations of black and foreign graduates in inner-city work, where enforcement resources are aimed against large providers and where practitioners may be most apt to feel the need—and possess the self-excusatory rationalizations—for cheating in order to compensate for the lower fees offered by Medicaid. Black physicians and foreign medical graduates may be more vulnerable to fraud detection because greater enforcement resources are focused on the communities in which they work.

Nationally, California accounted for forty-one sanctioned doctors (28 percent of the total), followed by New York with twenty-five (17 percent). Thereafter came Maryland with eight, Florida and Pennsylvania with seven each, Texas with six, and Michigan with five. These states have the largest Medicaid budgets, so their share of violators is not disproportionate.

Family or general practitioners accounted for the greatest percentage of violators (27 percent), followed by psychiatrists (18 percent), general surgeons (11 percent), internists (8 percent), and obstetricians and gynecologists (7 percent). The "other" category includes specialties with only one or two offenders. General practitioners, the largest category of sanctioned physicians, also represent the largest specialty in the profession. In contrast, psychiatrists were overrepresented among sanctioned physicians, partly because of their vulnerability to enforcement. Psychiatrists' bills are based on the time actually spent with patients. It is difficult for them to bill for extra services or interventions, but it is easy to "inflate" the time they spend with patients. The "time game" proves to be irresistible to some members of the profession, and the relative ease of catching them often induces enforcement authorities to focus resources on psychiatrists' Medicaid fraud. Anesthesiologists can also play the time game, but the time they are engaged with patients before, during, and after surgery is much more difficult to monitor. The disproportionate number of psychiatrists sanctioned for Medicaid offenses, however, cannot be laid solely at the doorstep of enforcement idiosyncrasies. Psychiatrists, as we shall see, have also been convicted of numerous other forms of illegal behavior.

We were also curious about whether women doctors were suspended from Medicaid in proportion to their presence in the profession. In the late 1970s and early 1980s about 10 percent of all physicians were women, and among the suspended doctors in our sample for whom we could ascertain gender, fourteen (about 10 percent) were women.

THE CRIMES

There are four basic categories of crimes committed by physicians caught violating Medicaid programs: (1) billing schemes, which include billing for services not rendered, charging for nonexistent office visits, or receiving or giving kickbacks; (2) poor quality of care, which includes unnecessary tests, treatments, and surgeries as well as inadequate record keeping; (3) illegal distribution of controlled substances, which includes drug prescriptions and sales; and (4) sex with patients whereby physicians, under the guise of "therapy," received payments for sexual liaisons with their patients. These categories are not mutually exclusive, and the latter two can also be regarded as subsets of poor quality of care.

Opportunities for Dishonesty

Opportunity is often the hallmark of white-collar crime by professional persons—a theme echoed by health care providers testifying before congressional committees. Two chiropractors convicted of Medicaid fraud maintained before a Senate subcommittee that the system was "so bad that it virtually invites" criminal activity.[1] A physician convicted of stealing several hundred thousand dollars from Medicaid and other government programs told a joint hearing of Senate committees that his criminal behavior was so flagrant that only a seriously flawed system could have permitted him to get away with what he did for so long. He testified that the forms he sent into the programs for payment were so "arrogant and outrageous" that the services could not possibly have been performed as he alleged they had been. He pointed out that the diagnoses he put down "didn't relate to either the services or to other diagnoses that were submitted at the same time."[2]

The fee-for-service nature of Medicaid payments provides dishonest doctors with ample opportunities to bill for services never rendered or rendered by others and to bill for unnecessary tests and procedures. At first, some Medicaid providers stumbled upon these possibilities. One physician, for example, tired of waiting for Medicaid payment, worried that the government might have lost his bills. He sent in duplicates and, in time, was paid twice. When such stories spread in the medical community, some doctors were convinced that "nobody was minding the store."

For other physicians, the opportunity to provide medical care without concern about the cost proved attractive bait for illegal behaviors. Under Medicaid's lax scrutiny, these physicians had only to convince themselves that certain services would benefit their patients, a conclusion made more appealing when the services also benefited the physicians' pocketbooks.

In the case files, we found numerous examples of reimbursements for patients who were never seen, double-billing for the same patient, billing for phantom services and lab tests, billing for fictitious visits to disguise illegal prescriptions for controlled substances, and "upgrading" services. Another scam, though one rarely treated as criminal fraud because of problems in proving intent, is billing for unnecessary services. Even surgeons who perform unneeded operations, which can be regarded as equivalent to assault, are rarely prosecuted unless the abuses are wanton, again largely because of the difficulty in second-guessing medical opinions and demonstrating recklessness or culpable intent.

Some physicians got into trouble when they billed Medicaid for services they erroneously thought were acceptable. An obstetrician, for example, was fined $5,000 and had to make restitution when he billed Medicaid for surgeries at which he was present but did not perform the operations. It had been "accepted and customary" in his private practice to charge an "appearance fee" for such services, and the doctor mistakenly thought he could bill Medicaid for his services as a "teaching physician."

Some billing schemes go undetected because government agencies fail to communicate with each other. One case involved a doctor who had graduated from Havana Institute just before Castro took power. On seven attempts she failed the Foreign Licensing Examination, so Illinois, where she was then living, decided to revoke her temporary license. Undaunted, she continued to practice and to bill Medicaid, which continued to pay her, unaware of the revocation of her license. Medicaid had reimbursed this doctor more than $180,000 before agents, investigating a pharmacy scam, discovered her because she also was involved in a scheme with the pharmacy owner. She diagnosed virtually all her patients as having an upper respiratory infection and prescribed an average of five to seven items. Most, such as soaps and shampoo, were medically unnecessary but were prescribed to benefit the pharmacy. The doctor cooperated with the Medicaid agents against the pharmacy owner and was allowed to plead guilty to one count of practicing medicine without a license. She was put on probation for a year.

Many illegal billing schemes probably go undetected because patients, other health care practitioners, and welfare workers have little to gain from reporting them; rarely do they become so incensed as to squeal on crooked providers. For example, of the 670 cases of misconduct reported in 1982 to New York State officials, only 33 came from hospitals and other health facilities, and 28 from other physicians. The officials said the overwhelming majority of cases were reported by the public, which the officials said was the least likely group to recognize a problem.[3] But some doctors were trapped after a person in the know provided the policing agency with inside information. Investigations of such cases can be planned carefully because the enforcement agents are likely to know what they are looking for before they begin. The following case is illustrative.

In November 1981 the San Diego Medi-Cal Fraud Unit received an anonymous phone call. The informant told the senior investigator that a National City physician was conspiring with welfare recipients to bilk the county's welfare program. The doctor would falsely certify individuals as medically disabled; in exchange, he would be paid cash or Medi-Cal coupons.

The investigating agent began by making a routine background check on the sixty-seven-year-old physician. It showed that his medical license was in good standing, that no malpractice suits had been brought against him, and that he was not in trouble with the California Department of Motor Vehicles. The investigator then turned to county welfare eligibility workers who might be familiar with some of the physician's patients. Agents usually interview the patients directly, but this investigator had been warned that some patients might be involved in the scheme.

The investigator found an eligibility worker who had a client who was a patient of the doctor. She described the client as "physically fit enough to play professional football." Yet each month for several years the doctor had certified this individual as disabled. The diagnosed disabilities included "angina pectoris, dislocation of the left shoulder, dislocation of the right shoulder, alcoholism, and organic brain disease."

With the assistance of an eligibility supervisor, the investigation unearthed two more social service workers who said their clients included welfare recipients whom this doctor monthly certified as disabled. What had aroused the workers' suspicion was that in each instance the doctor diagnosed the recipients as suffering from a different disability. Phone calls from the supervisor to other welfare workers then uncovered an avalanche of questionable diagnoses by the doctor. The investigator wrote:

She and her co-workers have suspected [the doctor] of wrongdoing for a long time. However, due to legal restraints they are unable to have the recipients examined by another doctor. They have based their suspicions on their observations of these recipients and numerous rumors passed on by other welfare recipients. . . . She has been told by other recipients that [the doctor] does not examine his patients and has gone as far as signing patient disability waivers in the office parking lot.

The investigator, perhaps out of civility or frustration, did not mention the eligibility workers' collective negligence in failing to report their suspicions to supervisors. Already overloaded with work, the welfare department employees were disinclined to cause trouble. But their silence cost taxpayers thousands of dollars.

The agent opened the paper-chase portion of his investigation by comparing the diagnoses listed on the welfare disability certifications with those the doctor had recorded for Medi-Cal payment. "The majority of the diagnoses differed or the dates of service were not the same," he wrote. The doctor's diagnoses for Medi-Cal billings showed some consistency. Patients with acute bronchitis in March, for example, had progressed in the doctor's diagnoses to emphysema by September. His diagnoses for the welfare department, however, varied wildly. A Medicaid "emphysema" patient was diagnosed during the same period on county welfare forms as having acute bronchitis, nervous disease, alcoholism, acute depression, infection of the right foot, and a lung infection.

Armed with this information and with the details the eligibility workers had supplied, the investigator authorized an undercover operation. On a January afternoon, an undercover agent approached the doctor's office:

She found the front door locked. The doctor answered the door and told her she had to wait outside until he could see her. Approximately one-half hour later she was allowed into the office. She found it to be extremely cluttered and filthy. She could not go in any further than the front door due to the debris. The doctor was eating tortillas he took out of the store wrapper, which he continued to eat during the duration of the visit.

She told the doctor she had been experiencing pain in her back since the end of November. She did not know the origin; however, she knew she hadn't sustained the injury from a fall. The doctor touched her back and then had her attempt a few knee bends. The examination lasted less than two minutes.

The doctor then asked her to have X rays taken and gave her a prescription for Valium. He also signed her one-month medical disability certification.

Since the visit had not turned up any criminal activity, the investigator returned to the paper chase and began studying the doctor's Medi-Cal billings for the previous summer. So far all he had were the eligibility workers' suspicions and some questionable diagnoses—not enough to indict the doctor, much less to convict him. The billing records, however, provided a nugget. During June and July the doctor had billed Medi-Cal twice a month for each of the 132 patients he claimed to have seen. It seemed very unlikely that a doctor would need to see every patient twice a month and that he would see the same number of patients from month to month.

The investigator planned another undercover operation, this time using an agent who feigned leg pain:

After a few questions concerning her leg problem, [the doctor] examined her legs and feet. The doctor filled out a form on which the agent saw two separate line entries on which the doctor had typed "examination and treatment." She signed this form in two places and observed [the doctor] place a Medi-Cal sticker on it. Less than two hours later, another operative was in the doctor's office: The doctor questioned him about his alleged condition. There was no physical examination other than the doctor held his hands. When he signed the Medi-Cal form, the doctor had only filled in the name at the top and left the remainder of the form blank. The doctor also signed the [disability certification].

Within weeks, the doctor had billed Medi-Cal for two visits by the first undercover agent. The investigator had continued to review the doctor's Medi-Cal claims and found that for two and a half years he "consistently billed and was paid two office visits per month for every recipient listed." During the period, he had collected $46,871 from Medi-Cal. Interviews with four patients who occasionally saw the doctor confirmed that he was double-billing. All denied seeing him twice in a month. Then records arrived showing that the doctor had double-billed for the final two undercover operations. That sealed his fate.

A felony complaint was filed charging eight counts of submitting fraudulent Medi-Cal claims. The physician pled not guilty, but three months later he agreed to plead guilty to a lesser charge, a misdemeanor of presenting false claims. The judge sentenced him to a $5,000 fine and ordered him to pay $30,000 restitution. In addition, he was ordered to withdraw from participation in Medicaid.

Doing Things His Way

The cases in which investigators had the easiest time demonstrating criminal intent began with personnel informing on their former employers, providing names, dates, and specifics of alleged wrongdoing and sometimes supplying records to support their allegations. The files do not show any instance of "whistle blowing"—informing on a current employer; in fact, current employees often attempted to hide or minimize their bosses' illegal activities.

The case of a Northern California physician is illustrative. Two former employees of the doctor contacted California's physician licensing board with reports of fraud less than a month after they left his employ. Both said they had attempted to cover for the doctor's crimes and to suggest to him that his actions were illegal. "It's my practice and my business, and I don't like anybody that is not submissive," the doctor had reportedly told one of the informants. Another former employee, who also provided damning testimony against the physician, told the authorities:

The doctor would not listen to her if she explained things that Medi-Cal would not permit. For example, she stated that circumcisions were not to be paid benefit of the Medi-Cal program and that this was explained to her by Medi-Cal. She tried to explain this to the doctor, but he always wanted to do things "his way." [The employee] quit the doctor's employ after nine months. Her reasoning was that she had "been treated like a slave" and was "fed up."

Perhaps this physician risked committing criminal acts because he believed his days as a doctor were numbered. A graduate of an overseas medical school, he had not obtained a California license until he was forty-five. Within three years, the licensing board had put him on ten years' probation. One year later, as the fraud unit opened its criminal investigation, the licensing board was moving to revoke his license.

Once, a former employee reported, the doctor had ordered her to bill for services a patient had refused. "Doctor," she told him, "if she complains about that, you're going to lose it altogether." The physician reportedly replied, "I don't care. I want what I can get out of it."

The doctor's criminal behavior was blatant and ubiquitous. He saw forty to fifty patients each morning at one office and then ten to twenty more at his afternoon office. Ninety percent of his practice was Medi-Cal. People might wait an hour to see him. He rarely set appointments, and he spent only a couple of minutes with a patient. Patients, it seems, appreciated his willingness to prescribe controlled substances. According to an informant, the doctor rarely examined a patient. "[He] would sit on the examining table and ask, 'What medicine do you want today?'"

The doctor maximized his Medi-Cal receipts by prescribing only enough medication to last two weeks and having patients return for a refill. The first visit was billed as an exam and the second as a recheck. Occasionally, patients returned for a third visit within a single four-week period. Because Medi-Cal does not routinely pay for three visits in one month on the same diagnosis, the doctor or his staff changed the diagnosis for the third visit and billed Medi-Cal for a new exam. The doctor sometimes arrived at the new diagnosis by asking the patient, "What else is wrong with you?"

The doctor did not even bother billing Medi-Cal for some procedures even though they were covered. Medi-Cal, for example, allowed estrogen injections once a month, but the doctor charged patients $9 a shot for all injections. He also charged Medi-Cal more than he did his few private patients. For example, he billed the program for $47 (although he was presumably reimbursed for less) for a "procedure" for which he charged his private patients $39. When told by one of his employees that such practices were not permissible, he "said he had to do it to balance out his books because Medi-Cal didn't pay enough."

The doctor also had a method for confiscating codeine from his patients:

[The informant] stated that when patients came for codeine, the doctor would phone the pharmacy for a prescription of 3 grains. . . . The pharmacy would automatically dispense sixty tablets. The patients did not want 3 grains; they wanted 4 grains. The patients would come back to the office with the vials of medication. The vials would be given to the receptionist, who gave the vials to the informant, who put the vials on the doctor's desk. The doctor put the vials in his desk drawer. He then called the pharmacy back with a prescription for 4 grains for the patient.

The second informant corroborated these details and added that the returned medications, as well as codeine samples, were taken home to the doctor's wife, who reportedly said, "I need it."

The doctor also routinely billed for services never rendered. One of the informants reported that he told his staff, "When a patient walks through the door, whether we do anything or not, you bill an office visit." The most glaring violation occurred when the doctor went to Las Vegas and ordered his unlicensed nurse to see patients, refill their medications, and bill as if he were present. This violation was the easiest for the prosecution to prove and, unlike most cases, it went to trial. The jury deliberated three hours before finding the doctor guilty of one count of grand theft for filing sixteen false claims. The judge sentenced the doctor to make restitution of $492, fined him $15,000, and ordered him to make his records available to Medi-Cal investigators so they might make additional recoveries. He also added five years' probation and 270 days in the county jail on a work furlough program. Under this program, the doctor would spend his days at his regular employment and his nights and weekends in jail. The judge allowed the convicted physician to spend the Christmas season at home; two weekends later the doctor had to report to the county jail.

Fake Laboratory Tests

Some physicians' employees accepted their bosses' illegal conduct in order to keep their jobs. The employee, in this regard, resembles the corporate criminal whose conduct mainly benefits the company. A deputy attorney general explained how he saw one such case:

The employee's conduct was inexcusable. However, her culpability is certainly not of the same character as the doctor's. It was the doctor whose orders she followed. As a physician and her employer, he occupied a position of leadership and dominance. Since the employee's only financial gain from this conduct was the job security that came from pleasing her employer, it is likely that the doctor's dominance was a significant factor in inducing her to participate in these misrepresentations.

This doctor had directed his employee of ten years to bill Medicaid for expensive office laboratory tests, although his patients actually received inexpensive tests performed by an outside laboratory. The doctor, a graduate of Harvard Medical School, had previously been in trouble: A decade earlier the state licensing board, citing his gross negligence in the treatment of pre- and postoperative patients and nursing home patients, had placed him on two years' probation and banned him from performing any major surgical procedures. Nine years later the board once again put him on probation, charging that he was excessively prescribing amphetamines and diuretics to patients with weight-control problems. The doctor pled guilty to grand theft from the Medicaid program; he still faced trial on charges that he had bypassed his home gas meter and unlawfully obtained $4,000 in gas to heat his swimming pool and spa.

The supervising deputy attorney general who prosecuted the case clearly wanted jail time for the doctor. He argued that the doctor's blatant criminal behavior had diverted funds from needy indigents and had contributed to the public's growing lack of confidence in the medical assistance programs. He added:

There is a prevailing perception that punishment for the poor is commonly more harsh than punishment for professionals such as the defendant. A visit to courtrooms throughout California will force you to conclude that the poor in our communities are routinely sentenced to county jail for theft offenses far less serious than the premeditated swindle at issue here.

I submit that the element of deterrence should be the most important factor considered by the court in imposing sentence in this case. Persons occupying positions of public trust are intelligent and capable of weighing the risks of detection and prosecution against the financial gain to be achieved by fraudulent conduct. Anything less than one year in county jail for a crime as socially reprehensible as this would only serve to encourage other persons in positions of public trust to steal from the public. The defendant should also be required to make [full] restitution. . . . Anything less will send a message to providers of the Medi-Cal program that crime can indeed pay. On the other hand, incarceration of the defendant as recommended will become known to other persons similarly situated and will constitute a deterrence that may tend to protect the public against millions of dollars in future losses from this billion-dollar program for the poor.

The judge agreed that the doctor should make full restitution but did not fine him, instead ordering one hundred hours of community service. There also was a sixty-day jail sentence.

Blowing the Whistle on Drug Dealing

Another case began with an informant's call to the Los Angeles County central fraud reporting line, a hotline established by the county's board of supervisors to receive fraud complaints, primarily welfare illegalities. The informant's taped message was short and to the point: "He's self-employed. He's an M.D., a family doctor. I'm calling because he is committing fraud against Medi-Cal. He's been lying about dates people come there, how long the patient stayed, diagnosis, and what they have done. I could give you specific information. I would like a response."

After a six-week delay, the message was forwarded to the state's Medicaid agency. An additional six months passed before an investigator interviewed this informant, a receptionist who had been fired for questioning the physician's billing practices. She told the investigator that the doctor charged for comprehensive exams that lasted only three minutes, that he routinely wrote prescriptions without examining patients, that urine samples were commonly taken and dumped without being analyzed, that electrocardiograms were given to all new patients but never read, and that many services were often billed but never provided.

The investigator decided to randomly select two of the doctor's Medi-Cal recipients for claims review. The review led the investigator to note that the "subject appears to be billing for an excessive amount of services." Nine months after the disgruntled former employee had telephoned the hotline, the case was referred to the MFCU for further investigation.

The MFCU already had an open file on the doctor when the health department's referral arrived. A month earlier it had received a complaint from the state licensing board. A patient had called the board to complain that the doctor had billed his insurance company for services not rendered. The licensing board, in its referral, noted it had attempted to stage an undercover operation but had been unable to locate an agent who matched the physician's clientele.

The criminal investigator opened the case and requested claims information. After reviewing the claims material, he began a series of interviews. Most patients reported that they saw the doctor twice a month and received prescriptions for codeine, Valium, and Darvon; some were given vitamin B-12 injections; others purchased diet pills that the doctor sold illegally. On their initial visit, the doctor took urine and often blood, and they were given an electrocardiogram. Subsequent office visits lasted from three to five minutes.

Often the prescriptions were not for the individual the doctor saw, but for another member of the family. One beneficiary stated that the only reason she saw the doctor was to obtain "codeine pills for her husband, who was suffering from a back injury, and was unable to see the doctor in person." The doctor, however, billed the benefit program for treating both the wife and husband. When a patient complained about becoming addicted to all the drugs the doctor prescribed, he told the patient to stop seeing him.

To cover his tracks, the doctor invented diagnoses. One patient, according to the bills, suffered from an airway obstruction, heart failure, bronchitis, neuralgia, neuritis, lumbago, and hypertension—all within a three-month span. The doctor also billed for injections he never gave, in one instance charging the government for two years of penicillin treatments for a patient who was allergic to the antibiotic.

The doctor also billed the government for "physical therapy," which lasted about five minutes and was given by his secretary. He asked some patients for two Medi-Cal stickers per visit, explaining that "one sticker is for the file and the other sticker is needed to submit to Medi-Cal for payment," and then billed Medi-Cal for two visits. The doctor's practices got patients into trouble with the health department, which restricted their Medi-Cal cards after it wrongly assumed that the "excessive visits" were their fault. The recipients, ignorant of the fake billings, never questioned the health department's decision. Most patients, however, were happy with the doctor's services; he gave them the drugs they wanted. Some traveled long distances to see him.

Twenty-two months after the former employee's telephone call, the doctor appeared in court for a preliminary hearing. Shortly thereafter, he pled guilty to three misdemeanor counts and was sentenced to five days in jail, five hundred hours of community service, and $6,000 in restitution. Two years after the initial complaint, during which time this doctor had received more than $100,000 in Medi-Cal payments, the health department put him on special claims review, which meant they would scrutinize his bills.

Another doctor prescribed controlled substances to alleged alcoholics without giving them a medical examination. He was charged with maintaining a business office for the purpose of prescribing drugs illegally. The doctor's doorman would control office traffic, screen patients to be sure they were not government agents, and collect $10 at the door before a patient would be waved in. The doctor also hired drivers to transport "patients" to his office. He was eventually convicted in a U.S. District Court jury trial for conspiracy for attempted distribution of controlled substances and for prescribing drugs without an examination. He was not charged with filing false Medicaid claims (although he had done so), but his conviction and thirty-month prison term led to his suspension from the Medicaid program.

In at least one case, a physician appears to have participated in an organized crime scheme. Five doctors and three pharmacists were among eleven persons convicted in a U.S. District Court for stealing about $20 million from the Illinois Medicaid program. They were accused of running a network of clinics, laboratories, and pharmacies that wrote and filled thousands of bogus prescriptions. The doctors had billed the Medicaid program for millions of dollars worth of unnecessary medical tests, examinations, and supplies. The fraud relied in part on the enlistment of physically and psychologically impaired doctors, some of them drug dependent. The clinics served only drug addicts, who paid cash for prescriptions in exchange for submitting to unnecessary tests and allowing a range of charges to be applied against their Medicaid cards. Whenever blood was drawn from one patient, the clinic billed the government for the taking and testing of blood from several patients. The government was also billed for items ranging from condoms to toothpaste. A government witness, a pharmacist who had pled guilty to charges of racketeering and mail fraud, was asked during the retrial of the doctor if the clinics ever treated any sick persons. "I hope not," he replied.

One of the clinic doctors had first gotten into trouble with the Illinois Medicaid program in 1969, a year after having been the program's highest-billing doctor in Chicago. He was suspended from Medicaid when it was discovered he was signing bills for care provided to Medicaid patients by another doctor who had been dropped from the program. But the ban was short-lived. Within months he was reinstated on the recommendation of the Cook County unit that managed the welfare program. In 1981, however, his name came up during an investigation of another doctor. Each of eight visits to the doctor's office by under-cover agents netted prescriptions for controlled substances—all without the legally required examinations. Noncontrolled substances were also freely prescribed. At each visit Medicaid patients were advised to pur-chase an average of ten to twelve items. One individual received twenty-nine items on a single service date, including rubbing alcohol and Phisohex.

The doctor steered patients to a pharmacy across the hall. In one year, the pharmacy received $516,000 in Medicaid payments from the state; 80 to 90 percent of the pharmacy's prescriptions were written by the doctor. It closed its operation within days of his indictment.

Over three years, this doctor personally had collected $300,000 from Medicaid. He was sentenced to thirty months' probation and was ordered to perform sixteen hundred hours of community service. The judge rejected the prosecutor's call for a prison term, saying that the doctor's abilities would be better utilized in service to the community.

Ironically, the doctor's attorney had argued to the judge that his client should be allowed to do public service work in lieu of prison because he was schizophrenic and under psychiatric care. The attorney also claimed that the doctor was "so passive at the time he committed the crimes that he would listen to and do anything anybody told him."

The Department of Registration and Education declared the doctor incapable of practicing medicine and prescribing drugs with reasonable safety and ordered his license suspended until he could prove that his medical condition had improved sufficiently for him to maintain "a minimum level of professional competency." This doctor's suspension lasted less than a year.

Medicaid and Murder

One of the most shocking Medicaid cases involved a physician living in Miami, Florida. She had arrived in the United States from Cuba in 1960 and claims to have graduated from medical school at the University of Havana. She began practicing medicine in Miami in 1967 while she completed her state licensing requirements. By 1980, five years after she began treating Medicaid patients, she had become the second largest provider of such services in Florida and was operating two clinics. According to official reports, she received $184,000 in state monies in 1980.

The doctor came to the attention of investigators when two women complained that her "acne treatments" had left them disfigured. In March 1981 the doctor was arrested on racketeering charges, which alleged that she had billed Medicaid for more than $97,000 for treatments never performed. During the jury trial, the prosecutor asked a witness if he had ever been treated by the doctor for acne, tonsillitis, viral fever, an ingrown toenail, depression, asthma, or diaper rash. The spectators and jurors laughed. The witness was a nineteen-year-old 220-pound college football player who had visited the doctor twice, complaining of a cold. But the doctor had billed the state for 51 visits and received payments of $1,885. Another of the ten witnesses testified that she had never even met the doctor, although the physician had used her Medicaid number to bill the state for 165 visits, totaling $1,638.

The jury took only one hour to convict the doctor on twenty-four counts of filing false claims and twenty-four counts of receiving payments to which she was not entitled. The judge sentenced her to twenty years in prison, saying, "This so-called white-collar crime is also stealing money allocated to the poor." A state attorney said that the money paid to the physician could have gone to treat more than ten thousand poor patients. The sentence was the most severe punishment yet given to a physician for Medicaid violations.

But the Miami doctor's story does not end here. Shortly after she was sentenced, she became a prime suspect in the murder of her former partner, who had been gunned down outside a Miami hospital a few weeks before the fraud indictment was announced. She was accused of having paid $10,000 for a contract killing to prevent her former partner from testifying against her in the fraud case.

During the murder trial, the prosecution produced a "hit list" containing the murdered partner's name and the name of the investigator heading up the case against the doctor. The doctor testified that the list was to be delivered to a *Santería* practitioner (*Santería* is a Caribbean religion) who had requested that she furnish names of people she might be involved with in future legal disputes. She did not believe in *Santería*, she said, but her accountant had recommended she try it to ease her mind.

The doctor was sentenced to life imprisonment with a twenty-five-year minimum sentence on the murder charge and another thirty years for conspiracy. The new sentences were to run consecutively with the twenty-year sentence she had already received for her Medicaid fraud conviction.

The convictions for conspiracy and murder were upheld in a district court of appeal, but on April 27, 1989, the Florida Supreme Court overturned the murder conviction and ordered a new trial. The court ruled that the circumstantial and hearsay evidence presented at the trial may have prejudiced the jury's decision.

Giving Birth to Gynecological Fraud

A California gynecologist came to the enforcement team's attention when the Surveillance and Utilization Review (SUR) unit of the state's health department routinely checked the records of the state's top two hundred providers. The files indicated that the doctor had billed Medi-Cal for analyzing Pap smears in his office when the analysis actually was done by an independent lab that charged less than half of what the government paid the gynecologist. In addition, the SUR investigators found evidence that he was double-billing the government for services.

This was not the first time the doctor had come to the attention of enforcement officials. A previous computer analysis had shown that he had billed for a variety of services with a frequency that far exceeded the average of providers of the same specialty in the same region. Health department investigators must have presumed the doctor was "up-grading" the office visits—charging for a more expensive procedure than the one actually performed—because they suggested he use a lower-paying billing code. But the doctor's billing pattern did not change.

When the SUR investigators forwarded the data they had collected to the Medi-Cal fraud unit, a criminal investigator there concluded that the doctor had altered information on billing forms "in an effort to get the claim through claims processing without being rejected. This appears to be a deliberate attempt to collect twice for the same procedures."

The investigator learned from the registered nurse who had performed the SUR investigation that the gynecologist did not have in his office the proper equipment to analyze Pap smears and that receipts in patient charts indicated the use of an outside lab—a matter the doctor admitted. A phone call to the lab revealed that the lab charged $3.50 for each Pap smear, for which the doctor billed Medi-Cal $8.40.

In total, the SUR investigation of eighty-five patient charts found

billing for procedures for which there was no record in the patient's chart: thirty patients, totaling fifty-three procedures, for $733.84

double-billing: seven patients, totaling ten procedures, for $1,054.70

billing for new patients who were actually established patients: two patients, totaling two procedures, for $51.22

billing for a circumcision for a female baby: one patient, for $23.40.

On the basis of this information, a judge issued a warrant to search the doctor's office and seize patient records and files. The doctor was visibly upset when he arrived at work to find half a dozen agents on hand. An investigator tape-recorded what followed and gave the following report, starting with the doctor's expression of indignation:

"I just really don't understand the Gestapo-like tactics of this, and you're welcome to any of my records, and this is ridiculous. To encroach upon my day, and embarrassment. I just don't think this is necessary." The agent began to tell the doctor, "If you have any questions—" The doctor interrupted, turned around, and faced the agent, his face being no more than twelve inches from the agent's face, and said, "I'm just telling you what I think. You listen for a minute. See, you're on my premises, you listen." The agent replied, "Sir, I am here under a court order to search your premises." The doctor stated, "That's fine, but this could have been carried out at another time. This is just absolutely ludicrous, and I deeply, deeply resent it. I think it's most inappropriate."

As the investigation continued, the agent discovered that the double-billings had been errors by the doctor's staff and that all duplicate payments from Medi-Cal had been routinely returned. Given that the doctor was billing Medicaid for amounts in excess of $150,000 a year, mistakes were inevitable. The evaporation of his best evidence, however, did not deter the investigator, who turned his attention to interviewing patients and employees.

The employees said that the doctor kept tight control on billing. After seeing a patient, he would list for the billing clerk what he had done and the charges. In such a large office, such attentiveness to each charge is unusual; most doctors leave such matters to their clerks.

The employees admitted they charged more than they paid for Pap smears but believed this was acceptable because, "as far as they understood it, the charge was for taking the Pap smear." The employees also described the office's standard procedure for billing for births: Bill for total obstetric care, spinal anesthesia, and newborn care; if the baby was a male, bill for a circumcision. Interviews with the doctor's patients, however, indicated they did not always have spinal anesthesia, and some had no anesthesia. One patient said that the doctor had given her two shots in the cervix while she was in labor, but "it wasn't like a spinal because they went up inside for the shot, and they don't for the spinal. The doctor asked what I wanted. He said if I took a spinal, I wouldn't feel any pain. I told him, 'No, I don't want one.'" As for the "newborn care," most patients were, understandably, unsure whether the doctor had examined their newborns as required for billing. They remembered he had looked at the babies and then given them to the nurses for cleaning.

When asked about office visits, patients were able to confirm that the doctor had submitted to Medi-Cal diagnoses of phantom illnesses, such as acute gastroenteritis, when they had gone for routine prenatal check-ups.

This gynecologist got into trouble in part because he followed his own whims in billing. He threw Medi-Cal update notices into the trash unread. He argued that he was entitled to higher pay for his office visits because he felt it necessary to have a nurse present during gynecological exams. He also believed he deserved the additional money he billed for Pap smears because he had to send the specimens to the laboratory and interpret the results—matters Medi-Cal deems covered by the cost of office visits.

Proving criminal intent in this case would not have been easy. The doctor was not without wile; for example, he erased a tape recording he had made of his initial meeting with the SUR investigators, probably because of telltale admissions. "I'm not as dumb as Nixon," he joked with the investigator when asked for the tape.

The government eventually chose to ignore the doctor's upgrading and billing for services not rendered and to concentrate solely on the Pap smear cases, which were the charges easiest to prove. On the billing form the doctor was supposed to check a box indicating where the Pap smear was analyzed. He usually failed to complete this item but had in some instances indicated that the work was done in his office. The prosecutors knew they had a solid case and charged the gynecologist with one count of grand theft and forty-one felony counts of filing false claims.

The doctor pled guilty to a negotiated charge of nine misdemeanor counts of filing false claims, but he maintained that "the violations were unintentional errors that occurred as a result of the complexities of the Medi-Cal billing system." The judge asked the doctor why he had pled guilty if he denied any criminal liability, and the judge then produced the Medi-Cal reimbursement form on which the doctor had indicated that the lab work was done in his office. He also pointed out that the doctor had billed for anesthesia that was never administered. The gynecologist was sentenced to repay $10,000, fined $5,000, and ordered to provide $10,000 in free obstetrical care to Medi-Cal patients at Medi-Cal rates.

Doctors in Large Clinics

The case files we reviewed included relatively few cases of doctors who used their corporate medical clinics to perpetrate fraud. The most likely explanation is that illegal billings can be hidden in a high-volume organization. Large-scale business not only provides dishonest individuals with camouflage for larceny but also allows them to place barriers between themselves and proof of their criminal culpabilities.

A Los Angeles physician who owned and operated a medical group billed Medicaid for his corporation's activities by using its Medi-Cal provider number. An investigation showed he routinely padded the bill by adding minutes to his group's charges for anesthesia services. A Los Angeles grand jury indicted the doctor on twenty counts of wrongdoing, but the prosecution ran into trouble when the district attorney's office realized that no law prohibited the doctor's behavior—a common oversight in the first decade of the benefit program. An agent wrote:

The whole case for fraud hangs on the doctor's misuse of time modifiers under the RVS [relative value scales—an insurance billing mechanism]. The problem is somewhat surprisingly that the RVS, although in common usage at the time, had never been adopted as a regulation of the Department of Health when the conduct in this case was occurring. Without undue elaborations, suffice it to say, there were serious legal problems of a due-process nature connected with penalizing anyone for breach of standards which are not a matter of written law. . . . If taken to trial, this case would be quite time-consuming, and the result would be difficult to predict.

Following heated pretrial arguments, the defense and prosecution struck a deal. A year and a half after the indictment, the doctor appeared in court to plead no contest to an amended charge of receiving stolen property. By agreement, his practice of medicine was put on probation for two years and he was ordered to provide 384 hours of community service during that period. In addition, the state's health department suspended him (and his corporation) from billing Medi-Cal for five years. An agent in the case wrote to the state's medical licensing board urging them to acquiesce in the agreement: "It is as tough a penalty as we would likely be able to achieve, even if we tried the case; it deters the doctor, it gives the board supervisory power over him for two years, and it will serve as a warning to other doctors."

Interjurisdictional Problems

Like many enforcement and regulatory officials, those concerned with Medicaid investigation and administration often feel frustrated by what they regard as judicial leniency and indulgence. Enforcement problems are multiplied in instances where suspect doctors move from one state to another. For example, a New York physician was convicted of stealing approximately $20,000 from the state's Medicaid program by billing for services he never performed. The court fined him $5,000, placed him on probation for three years, and ordered him to complete a one-year obligation as a VISTA volunteer. After the New York conviction, California routinely revoked this physician's license to practice medicine in that state. (Doctors frequently hold licenses in more than one state.) The doctor's request for reinstatement tried to dispel his criminal image:

He is a board-certified pediatrician, and is employed as a pediatrician on the poverty program operated in New York City by the neighborhood health services program. Throughout his medical career, the doctor has demonstrated a continuing interest in, and commitment to, the development and implementation of community health care programs. He provides medical supervision to . . . a settlement house in New York City founded in 1889 which serves preschool children, adolescents, and senior citizens primarily from minority, low-income families living in Manhattan. He has served as a VISTA volunteer and worked with the federal Headstart Health Care Program. He also serves as a pediatrics lecturer for the Stony Brook Physician Assistant Program operated by the State University of New York. He is aware of the serious nature of his misconduct and is contrite. There is no evidence of any other criminal activity before or since the conduct in question, which occurred approximately seven years ago. The doctor appears to have rehabilitated himself. He is in compliance with all terms and conditions of the orders of probation.

One member of California's licensing board was dismayed by the doctor's dossier and commented, "He can stay in New York. I cannot believe the double standard concerning physicians. If some middle-class or poor person had committed the same crime, they would be in prison. Are the judges protecting doctors? Maybe we should do something. I realize this happened in New York, but we have had similar cases here—$20,000 stolen, $5,000 returned. Question: Is this rehabilitation?" Doctors convicted of serious offenses can often resurrect their practices elsewhere. This doctor was not relicensed in California. However, other states are not so strict in preventing errant physicians from practicing within their boundaries.

THE PUNISHMENTS
The Judicial Response

The records we reviewed do not enable us to draw definitive conclusions about judges' attitudes toward errant doctors. But it appears that judges do make an effort to tailor sentences to fit what they perceive as the special conditions of convicted doctors. For example, a psychiatrist who routinely billed the government for services either not rendered or rendered by others could have been held to account for up to $360,000—$260,000 for overcharges, $37,000 in interest, and $62,000 for government investigative costs. When the psychiatrist pleaded guilty to one felony count of grand theft, the court placed him on eight years' probation, ordered him to pay a $5,000 fine and to make restitution of $160,000, and sentenced him to six months in a county work furlough program that allowed him to work during the day but spend his nights in jail. The judge also offered the doctor the opportunity to reduce the restitution by up to $50,000 by providing a thousand hours of community service—a pay scale, $50 an hour, far higher than Medi-Cal rates at the time.

The psychiatrist probably did not deserve such special treatment. Only one month before his sentencing, he was still cheating the government. When he told a patient that "he was going to get his money one way or another," the patient complained to the government. Fifteen months later, the state Medicaid agency forwarded to the MFCU a file its agents had compiled on the doctor based on this complaint. The chief of the MFCU was shocked to find the new information unattached to the main case file. A few phone calls revealed the cause. A "computer misplaced the civil case," she was told.

Medical Mercy

Another case that illustrates the leniency accorded to high-status offenders is that of a fifty-year-old Brooklyn internist who had been paid $250,000 by Medicaid. This doctor had consistently billed for office visits, injections, and electrocardiograms he never performed. Before fraud charges could be brought, a federal grand jury indicted him on fifteen felony counts of narcotics distribution and sales. He consented to plead guilty to two counts and went to jail for four months; his medical license was revoked. When he was released from jail, the state charged him with 137 acts of Medicaid theft; he pled guilty to 3. The judge, in sentencing him to a conditional discharge, noted the doctor's recent incarceration on the unrelated offenses and his loss of license. The fact that the doctor was nearly destitute also contributed to the judge's decision to be merciful. It is unlikely that a poor person with a previous conviction for narcotics sales would have been treated so indulgently.

Revoking Licenses

It is unusual for physicians to lose their medical licenses for Medicaid violations. During the first eight years of the program, California routinely lifted the California licenses of doctors sanctioned in New York but pulled the license of only one of its own Medicaid violators. The case of that doctor, a psychiatrist, illustrates how only the most egregious violations get a doctor booted out of medicine.

The psychiatrist first ran into trouble with the Medicaid program over hundreds of bills for psychiatric treatments she never rendered. The case relied heavily on the testimony of owners and administrators of nursing homes. After a year's delay, however, some witnesses were not as sure as they originally had been about the doctor's failure to provide psychiatric care.

Because of the ambiguities in the witnesses' testimony, the state's licensing board concluded it was best to seek a negotiated penalty. An agreement was reached by which the psychiatrist received five years' probation and a nine-month suspension of her license. She also was required to provide eight hours of free community service a week for the first year and four hours a week for the remaining four years of probation. Even during the nine-month suspension, she was allowed to practice medicine as long as her work was limited to community service. The board noted, "The variation in the standard form of this condition seems justified as the public will derive some benefit from her activities. We have no evidence that she is unqualified, from a clinical standpoint, to practice medicine."

Less than a year later, the board acted to revoke the psychiatrist's license permanently. During a few morning hours over eighty days of working at a clinic in a building she and her husband owned, she had written twenty-eight hundred prescriptions, most of them for controlled substances such as Ritalin, Valium, and codeine, which she would prescribe without examinations. She also failed to fulfill most of the conditions of her probation.

In contrast to California's board, which automatically revokes the license of any doctor convicted of a crime in another state lest California become a retreat for wayward doctors, Georgia's board appears less willing to issue revocations or suspensions. A Georgia doctor convicted of twenty-three felonies for filing false claims was suspended from practice for three months and given five years' probation. In several states, including California, New York, and New Jersey, doctors can expect major license troubles if convicted of even one felony.

Georgia's judiciary also seems to be lenient with doctors who file false claims. One physician fraudulently billed the state's Medicaid program for $13,000. He was allowed to plead no contest to a misdemeanor. The court fined him $1,000 to be paid, with interest at 7.5 percent, at $85 a month. He was put on probation until he finished paying the fine.

The state licensing board also placed him on probation for three months.

Judges are not inclined to send doctors to prison for billing for services never rendered. Again and again they assign probation and community service in lieu of suspended prison terms. The files we saw did not indicate the judges' sentencing criteria. The two rationales that seem most likely are that stealing funds from a government program is deemed similar to a property offense (first-time thieves are rarely sent to prison) or that physicians are too valuable a community resource to waste in prison.

Consider a New Jersey physician who pled guilty to a twenty-count indictment of Medicaid fraud. The behaviors charged represented only the tip of the doctor's criminal activities, evidenced by his repayment to the state of $60,000 in addition to a $30,500 fine. The judge sentenced the doctor to twenty years in prison but immediately suspended the prison term in favor of "two days per week gratuitous service at a hospital." The president of the New Jersey Medical Licensing Board, which revoked the doctor's license, took a firmer stand:

The illegal conduct was a systematic pattern which persisted over a three-year period. . . . Further, while letters on behalf of the doctor describe him as the only dermatologist serving a poor population in Newark, it is notable that the conduct for which he was convicted arose out of treating that same population which he now argues could benefit by his continued licensure. His crime shook public confidence in the Medicaid system as well as having attempted to divert public dollars. Despite attempts to characterize defendant's conduct as a mere digression from an otherwise virtuous life, there exists a wide gap between this individual's conduct and that which the public has a right to expect from a physician.

In another case, the New Jersey Medical Licensing Board also rejected a doctor's appeal for leniency based on his long list of good deeds: "That those anti-social activities continued concurrently with respondent's charitable work in no way lessens the breach of public trust committed by respondent under the privileged mantle of his medical licensure. Clearly, he utilized the privilege of his title to perpetrate the fraud and hoped to elude detection by the well-publicized acts of good works."

Negotiated Administrative Settlements

Sanctioned physicians face punishments from Medicaid administrators (suspensions and restitution), criminal courts (jail, fines, restitution), and physician licensing boards (license suspensions, revocations, fines). So at times physicians choose to negotiate settlements with enforcement officials and thereby possibly avoid criminal and licensure actions. Negotiations often result in voluntary, permanent suspensions from Medicaid and large restitutions. New York's Medicaid agency, for example, charged a physician with negligence and incompetence and ordered him to repay $32,000. The doctor agreed to withdraw voluntarily from the state's assistance program, and the Medicaid agency agreed to "withdraw its allegations of unacceptable practices" and to stipulate that the doctor "in no way admits to any wrongful intent or unlawful acts nor shall there be deemed such wrongful intent or unlawful acts in connection with such withdrawal from the program." After such an agreement, neither the state medical board nor a criminal court could use the administrative settlement as a basis for further action.

Such negotiated agreements between crooked doctors and the state's Medicaid agency were common in New York, probably because the agency appeared to be lenient, particularly when a physician compared the proposed administrative sanctions to the potential sentence for a criminal conviction.

New York State routinely audits its highest-billing Medicaid providers, believing that a doctor can see only so many Medicaid patients in a year and those who greatly exceed the norm are most likely to be using fraudulent tactics. Besides, only a big biller can be stealing a substantial sum; a physician who has a small Medicaid practice could not be cheating on a large scale.

For each of these high-billing doctors, the department selects a statistically valid sample of patient case files. In one instance, 100 cases were chosen from 3,327 Medicaid patients and a $157,000 billing to represent twenty-six months of a physician's practice. When this doctor was unable to produce charts for 36 of the cases, investigators discovered numerous deficiencies in his records and quality of care. Extrapolating from the sample to the doctor's full caseload, the auditors estimated that the doctor owed Medicaid $72,000 plus $6,000 interest. The agency and the doctor negotiated a settlement that included restitution of part of the estimated theft and a delayed voluntary permanent withdrawal from the state's welfare programs.

The files of negotiated settlements contain some agreements that seem unsettling given the scope and seriousness of the physicians' crimes. One audit, for example, concluded that half of one doctor's $240,000 Medicaid payments were illegally obtained. Further, it revealed:

(a) the consistent failure to provide adequate histories (e.g., presenting symptoms, complaints) to pursue diagnosis; (b) physical examinations, necessary for information indispensable to good medical care, which are incomplete, illegible or absent and are never directed by historical findings; (c) radiographs and electrocardiographs which are not interpreted or are inadequately interpreted; (d) diagnoses which are inconsistent with history, examination or lab findings, or which are not stated at all; (e) the consistent failure to record dates, treatment plans or dispositions; (f) the prescription of medications inappropriate or without regimes; and (g) the overutilization of psychotropic drugs.

Yet the state agency negotiated an agreement in which the total claim against the doctor was $77,000, and the agency agreed to accept $59,000 to be paid over two years with interest. The doctor's voluntary permanent suspension was delayed six weeks, during which time he was paid half of any Medicaid funds he earned, with the other half credited to his restitution.

Doctors who faced criminal procedures prior to Medicaid administrative actions fared worse than those who took their Medicaid lumps first. The criminal procedures usually resulted in lower restitution orders, but the doctors were suspended from Medicaid and faced licensure actions as well as adverse publicity—penalties avoided by doctors who agreed to negotiated settlements.

Some physicians convicted of crimes fight subsequent civil and administrative actions. A plea of no contest in a criminal action, for example, was later used by a doctor at an administrative hearing to try to block further action. At the hearing to bar him from Medicaid, he argued that he had no criminal intent and that his no contest plea was entered to avoid the possible adversities of going to trial. The prosecutor noted that a plea of no contest, according to court decisions, was to be accepted only when there was a "strong factual basis for the plea." The doctor also contested his permanent suspension from Medicaid on the grounds that he had cooperated with prosecutors and because "he previously enjoyed a good reputation in his community and profession." The prosecutor, in rebuttal, stated the government's position on suspension from Medicaid:

Appellant's cooperation and previous good reputation do not relieve the State of its obligation to exclude from participation in the Medical Assistance program providers whose conduct constitutes an unacceptable practice. Appellant knowingly and repeatedly defrauded the Medical Assistance program and can no longer be trusted as a provider in that program. Furthermore, it should be remembered that participation in the Medical Assistance program is voluntary and contractual in nature. No vested right is being denied the provider, as would be the case if an unacceptable practice hearing could result in a criminal conviction or in the revocation of the provider's license to practice his profession. Since the relationship between provider and government agency is a voluntary and contractual one, that government agency should have wide latitude in deciding which providers it will do business with.

Drugs, Sex, and Psychiatrists

Fraud by Psychiatrists. As noted earlier, psychiatrists were over-represented in our sample of doctors who committed Medicaid fraud. The most common offense was inflating the amount of time spent with patients. There are also cases of billings for fictitious patients and for therapy administered by someone other than the psychiatrist. Psychiatrists have also been caught dispensing drugs to patients and charging the government for therapy time. They have also become involved sexually with patients or former patients and have billed the benefit program for such dalliances.

As discussed earlier, what is known and believed about fraud against government medical benefit programs by psychiatrists reflects particularly unfavorably on them. But there is extenuating evidence suggesting that the high rate of fraud by psychiatrists, compared with that of physicians in other specialties, may be a function of their particular susceptibility to discovery and successful prosecution. Consider, for example, the differences between psychiatrists and anesthesiologists, specialists who also bill for the time spent with patients rather than for specific procedures. Unlike the psychiatrist's patients, the anesthesiologist's patients are in no condition during treatment to remember the duration of the physician's activities. Nor do anesthesiologists have much opportunity to become familiar with patients or to exchange drugs for payment or sex. Investigators must rely almost entirely on checking hospital records concerning the times of surgeries as well as established billing norms of anesthesiologists in order to convince a prosecutor to bring charges. As a result, the behavior of an anesthesiologist who inflates his record may surface only during a routine audit and investigation—a rare occurrence.

As to the issue of billing for work done by others, one must consider that various professionals bill for services performed by their staffs. Lawyers, for instance, often charge their clients high hourly fees for work performed by low-paid clerks. Medicaid, however, views such activities by doctors as an abuse of the program. And overwhelmingly it is psychiatrists who are caught billing for others' work, although various physicians have been sanctioned for such billing. For example, two doctors got into trouble when they submitted bills for supervising hearing exams at which they were not present, and another physician billed Medi-Cal for X rays he claimed were taken in his office under his supervision, though they were actually taken by unauthorized personnel in a different city.

When psychiatrists have had sex with patients and charged the government for therapy, the sexual misconduct has overshadowed the issue of fraud, which was usually viewed as a minor aspect of the case. All but one of the sex cases in the files we analyzed involved psychiatrists. The intense intimacy that can develop between doctor and patient is unlikely to occur nearly as readily in other specialties. A case that involved an osteopath seems almost childlike compared to the instances of psychiatric sexual abuse. The osteopath admitted to having felt the breasts of four female patients and having kissed three of the four without their consent. He pled guilty to four counts of sexual abuse in the third degree and was disqualified from the state's Medicaid program.

Psychiatrists often got into trouble with Medicaid because the autonomy they enjoy as independent providers of service runs afoul of Medicaid regulations. One clinician, for example, was suspended from Medi-Cal because he had charged the program for group psychotherapy sessions at which he was not present and that were led by his wife, a psychiatric nurse. He said the patients were told that his wife was a psychiatric nurse and not a physician, and that he and his wife discussed the cases after the sessions. Since his wife was a psychiatric nurse and provided the group psychotherapy under his supervision, he felt that he qualified as the provider for billing Medi-Cal.

Another psychiatrist was caught because his billings for the year were astronomical; he had billed for psychotherapy services rendered by nonlicensed personnel, including one individual who was a linoleum salesman when he was not delivering "psychotherapy." When the psychiatrist learned he was being investigated, he hired the former director of the state's MFCU, an attorney, to defend him. Before long, the psychiatrist skipped town and phoned another psychiatrist to persuade him to remove damaging files from his office. The colleague instead called the MFCU and told them about the files. The suspected psychiatrist eventually pled guilty.

Dishonest psychiatrists have victimized employees as well as patients and the government. One psychiatrist who charged the government for sessions provided by psychologists and nurses repeatedly promised his employees a percentage of the payments but often failed to make good. He promised a nurse 50 percent of what Medi-Cal offered, but she quit after repeated problems in collecting her salary. Another nurse left because the psychiatrist was using the payroll money for a Hawaii vacation—something he had done before. The nurse and others turned him in to the labor board and collected what was owed them. As if this were not enough, the psychiatrist was receiving a 10 percent kickback from another psychiatrist to whom he was referring cases.

Apparently, some doctors believed that even the most blatant cheating would go undetected. As early as 1969, one psychiatrist had habitually billed Medi-Cal for one-hour psychotherapy sessions that were at most half-hour visits or totally nonexistent encounters. Between May 1977 and July 1977, he billed Medi-Cal for twenty-four to twenty-eight individual one-hour sessions on each of eight separate days. On one "twenty-six-hour day," he billed an additional ten hours for private patients, producing a thirty-six-hour billing day. It was simple for the investigators to choose a couple of the doctor's more astonishing days (twenty-seven and twenty-eight hours billed) and to interview the beneficiaries the doctor claimed to have treated.

When the investigator went to the psychiatrist's office with a search warrant to seize records, the psychiatrist's lawyer was there and refused to allow the investigator to question his client. The lawyer argued that it was common for doctors to inflate time "to receive comparable payments as they receive from private patients," and he attempted to derail criminal prosecution by offering to have the doctor repay any illegal bills. "Hypothetically speaking," the lawyer offered, "if 40 percent of the total amount the doctor received from Medi-Cal were returned, would this stop any criminal action?" At his jury trial, the psychiatrist was represented by a different lawyer, but the 40 percent estimate of overpayment his first attorney had suggested came back to haunt him when the government used that figure to estimate restitution at about $125,000.

Before the trial, the doctor had removed his appointment books for prior years from his office. A search warrant for his home produced the books, which constituted the only record of the therapy sessions for the times in question. Some of the pages were missing, but these reappeared during the trial with numerous erasures, additions, and alterations in handwriting different from that of the doctor's secretary. The doctor admitted taking the appointment books but denied they had been altered. His secretary said that she could not explain the erasures. The psychiatrist denied telling a former patient, who was called to testify, to "be evasive" and to claim that some of her sessions were forty-five minutes long. The doctor maintained the witness had "hallucinated the event." He also denied telling a patient he was reducing her sessions to one-half hour because Medi-Cal would no longer pay for one-hour sessions. As justification, the doctor stated at his trial, "The traditional model of psychotherapy was put together . . . for affluent or middle-class patients. They can afford it, and they're verbal, articulate. Poor people aren't like that. They're often nonverbal. You can't have them talk for fifty minutes."

During the trial, according to the deputy attorney general, the psychiatrist continued to deny, minimize, and rationalize his guilt, blaming former secretaries for his difficulties. His attorney contended that the rules governing Medi-Cal billings were contradictory and confusing, that the errors were unintentional. The doctor's wife, who was his bookkeeper, testified that her husband worked seven days a week, got up before dawn, labored until 11 P.M. or 2 A.M., and answered telephone calls from patients at all hours of the night. Despite her testimony, her husband was convicted of one count of grand theft and eighteen counts of Medi-Cal fraud. The conviction, however, was not easily won. A second trial was ordered after the jury, following a twelve-day trial and two and a half days of deliberation, split 9–3 in favor of conviction. The second trial lasted four weeks, but this second jury took only two and a half hours to find the psychiatrist guilty. The doctor was not there to hear the verdict. The judge, rather than immediately issuing a bench warrant, as is typical when a "common" criminal fails to show, gave the psychiatrist until 9 o'clock the next morning to appear.

The prosecutor had argued for a prison term and was disappointed when the psychiatrist was sentenced to six months in jail and ordered to pay a $5,000 fine and make restitution. He was also suspended from government health programs for seven years. Although he received an unusually heavy sentence, the psychiatrist retained the real estate portfolio he had acquired—quite likely using Medi-Cal money: fifteen parcels whose tax assessment value was $1.4 million (the market value would have been much higher).

Another psychiatrist billed for patients he never saw. He would tell a mother that he needed Medi-Cal stickers for all her children even though he provided therapy for only one. He also obtained Medi-Cal stickers for canceled appointments. Investigators were tipped off by a patient who received a notification of benefits and observed that the doctor had billed for services rendered while the patient was in jail. An undercover operation and interviews with other beneficiaries quickly unearthed additional fraudulent bills. The doctor's billing clerk explained that if patients saw the doctor more than eight times in four months (Medi-Cal's limit without prior authorization), the billings were spread over a longer period to meet the legal requirement. When the investigator stated that such practices were illegal, the clerk replied that the procedure was intended only to help the patients.

In another case, a computer review revealed that a psychiatrist billed for eighteen patients in one day, all of whom he diagnosed as suffering from "anxiety neurosis." Investigator interviews with the doctor's patients indicated that he was billing for psychotherapy on patients whom he treated for general medical disorders such as diabetes and arthritis. The psychiatrist had billed Medi-Cal for scores of therapy sessions that he had not provided and that he claimed were performed in a health center where he was a salaried employee.

This doctor learned he was under investigation when one of his patients informed him that she had been interviewed by the fraud unit. He contacted a lawyer friend and asked him to intercede. The lawyer met with the fraud unit investigator and stated that the doctor wished to repay the $29,000 he had stolen. But the investigator continued his inquiries, noting that the doctor's provider number was "littered with fraud." These ongoing interviews prompted a phone call from the psychiatrist's attorney, who said he was worried that the investigation "was creating a potential problem" for the doctor with regard to his patients.

The doctor's admission of guilt and desire to repay the government probably did not work to his advantage. The government investigator had decided to end the investigation after uncovering $3,500 in fraudulent payments. The judge who sentenced the doctor, however, ordered him to make restitution of $29,000—the figure first supplied by the doctor—and fined him $5,000. The doctor's admission of guilt prior to any plea agreement made it easier for the prosecutor to obtain a ninety-day jail sentence.

The Medicaid fraud files show several other cases in which psychiatrists attempted to use the "patients' health" to deter further investigation. One psychiatrist's attorney wrote the head of the state fraud unit about the doctor's concern that "the mental health of the patient can be impaired by heavy-handed examination by your staff." The psychiatrist had informed his attorney "that the psychological condition of a number of his patients has deteriorated as a direct result of the contacts."

He suggested to the chief enforcement agent "that any further contact between his patients in your office either be supervised by [me] or be made by a board-certified psychiatrist with sufficient experience in handling chronic psychotic patients to minimize the potential for damage."

Out of Retirement and into Trouble.   The rationalizations offered by another delinquent psychiatrist illustrate a perverse form of professional jealousy. This psychiatrist had retired in his mid-sixties, when the state mental institution where he worked was closed. Friends, however, convinced him to come to work with them at a clinic in a poor neighborhood. They would provide him with an office, free of charge, the services of the clinic's receptionists, and a steady supply of referrals. As the psychiatrist later told investigators:

A number of my friends, who were GPs and had a clinic in the ghetto area, told me to come on down. They had a need for psychiatrists. These people who lived in the ghetto area were reluctant to travel to the then state hospital outpatient treatment service or the county hospital outpatient treatment service, so they were not being treated. And, rather reluctantly, I went down and began to enlarge my practice. Like Topsy, it grew awfully fast, and it became a very busy place. . . . The practices of the GPs and the dentist in the building were conducted essentially like a county hospital outpatient spot. It was thronged. People would drop in from all over: babies crying, milk bottles strewn on the floors, kids screaming, sick people, accident cases being brought in. It was a very, very busy place. The doctors referred many of the psychiatric people to me.

The doctor's trouble began when he continued to practice after his health failed. Instead of retiring, he lessened the time he spent with patients, eventually merely renewing their prescriptions. Almost all of his patients were Medi-Cal recipients, and he always billed the program for therapy hours. He also billed for missed visits, charged for individual psychotherapy for sessions provided to a family as a group, charged office visits for prescription refills, and prescribed medications for patients who had no pathology and whom he had not examined. Among his most serious offenses was the indiscriminate prescribing of Ritalin, a drug that calms hyperactive children but acts as a strong stimulant in adults. The doctor, however, ignored the question of how to treat young adults and prescribed Ritalin for four siblings, aged nineteen, seventeen, thirteen, and twelve.

Among the numerous rationalizations this psychiatrist provided for his behavior was the complaint that he could not bill the way the general practitioners did: "I was running an outpatient clinic just as well as the other doctors in the building. Only I would stay later, and I would come in earlier because these guys could do a one-minute thing, even a new patient, and order the bronchitis medicine, or whatever, unless it was a more serious thing. Yet, I couldn't do that sort of thing."

Inappropriate Psychiatric Treatment.   In another case, a psychiatrist was one of three responsible for treating 180 patients at a residential institution for the extremely mentally ill. Psychotherapy was not appropriate for most of the patients, whose average attention span was less than fifteen minutes, according to one nurse. Another nurse described seven of the patients in the following terms:

(1) almost a vegetable; no conversation, is dangerous; (2) curses, loses his temper easily, has a one-track mind; (3) a mute, does not talk; (4) a nonfunctioning person, asks, Where is my room? Is it smoking time? Is it time to eat?; (5) responds to conversation by saying his legs are cut off, won't let anybody touch him; (6) will not talk, walks away, pushes the doctor away when he tries to hang onto him; (7) slow-motion person, walks away.

Some of the patients could handle short therapy sessions, but only a handful received much therapy. Usually the psychiatrists simply reviewed the medical charts and adjusted medications.

When one of the psychiatrists realized that an investigation was being conducted at the institution, he approached the agent and asked about his status. The investigator, at the institution to investigate two doctors who had worked there before and had used a similar scheme, originally had not been interested in the psychiatrist, but his name had come to the agent's attention by accident while he reviewed institutional records. The agent told the psychiatrist he was being criminally investigated and read him his *Miranda* rights. The psychiatrist immediately admitted guilt and provided details of his crimes: He usually saw thirty patients in one day and billed for thirty hours of therapy, spread over several days. He also admitted that one month he became frightened and cut his billings. He hoped his cooperation would lead to a minimal punishment—the repayment of fraudulent gains.

Eventually this psychiatrist pled guilty to one count of grand theft and agreed to make restitution of $9,000. The probation officer writing the presentence report included a favorable report from the investigator regarding the doctor's cooperation. The psychiatrist was also sentenced to 30 days in jail, to be served on weekends, and 350 hours of community service.

Determining the Take.   Estimating the amount of money a doctor has stolen from Medicaid was important to investigators, who needed such figures to determine the extent of court-ordered restitution and to convince prosecutors to take a given case. Auditors often extrapolate years' worth of phony bills from average daily figures. This practice is not accepted by all criminal courts, but when it is allowed, it saves immeasurable hours of tedious work. For example, a psychiatrist who billed the government for therapy sessions conducted by a clinical psychologist and a social worker in his employ came to the government's attention because of his excessive billings. The auditor scrutinized one month of Medicaid payments made to the doctor in each of three years. He then subtracted legitimate payments from that total and divided the remainder by the number of working days in the period to establish an average daily loss. The psychiatrist was ordered to repay about $140,000 to the state. His attorney proposed he sell his half-million-dollar home and use the proceeds to pay his legal fees and part of the restitution. When the psychiatrist extended financing to the buyers, the auditor complained that the doctor stood to make a profit because the interest rate he was charging the buyers exceeded the rate the state was charging him on the balance of his restitution. So, a deal was struck by which the loan payments were sent to the probation department instead of to the psychiatrist.

Oral Copulation as Therapy.   In the case files we also found reports of psychiatrists who had sexual contact with patients. How prevalent is sexual misconduct? In a survey answered by 1,314 psychiatrists in 1986, 7 percent of the male psychiatrists and 3 percent of the female psychiatrists said they had had sexual contact with a patient. Moreover, 65 percent of these psychiatrists said they had seen at least one patient who reported sexual contact with a previous therapist; only 8 percent had reported these cases to authorities.[4]

When investigators suspect a doctor of patient abuse, they cannot rely on a paper trail that can be introduced at a trial to convince jurors of a defendant's guilt. Instead, they typically must stage an undercover operation. The following case illustrates some of the difficulties they encounter.

A psychiatrist came under investigation when a patient turned first to health administrators and then to the local police. She said she had begun to see the doctor seven years earlier because she had been depressed over her recent divorce. The doctor gave her tranquilizers and sleeping aids on the first visit. By her third session, she felt she was becoming dependent on the drugs, and she acquiesced to the doctor's request that she have oral sex with him. For the next seven years, she continued to see him on a monthly basis: she would perform fellatio, and he would write drug prescriptions for her.

The state licensing board's review unearthed two other patients who claimed similar experiences. The board assigned an investigator and an undercover operative to run a "sting" on the psychiatrist. The agent, equipped with a hidden microphone, saw the doctor and complained that she was depressed over her separation from her husband. What follows are excerpts from the investigator's report:

He repeatedly returned to the subject of conversation regarding the patient's sexual activity, asking her such questions as whether or not she masturbated or whether she has ever had a climax while she was sleeping. The doctor ultimately stated that one of her problems was that she had a cold, unemotional relationship with her father and, subsequently, married her husband subconsciously looking for a father figure. After approximately forty minutes, the doctor gave the agent a capsule which he wanted her to take. He stated the capsule would relieve the tension in her stomach. When the doctor turned his back, the agent dropped the capsule into her purse.

[At the end of the session] the psychiatrist gave her prescriptions for an antianxiety and antitension pill as well as one for an antidepressant. A week later the agent returned. The conversation, which lasted approximately one hour, dealt mainly with the agent's marital and sexual problems. The doctor stated the agent subconsciously wanted to have a sexual relationship with her father. During the conversation the doctor continually changed all subjects back to sex and, on a couple of occasions, asked the agent if she had sexual fantasies about him. The doctor stated, this feeling for a doctor by a patient does occasionally happen. The doctor persistently talked about whether or not the agent could have a sexual relationship with him and, at one point, asked if she felt that if she had sex with him it would be a gratifying experience.

Shortly thereafter, the agent returned to the office to take two personality tests, but she did not see the psychiatrist. Two days later she came back for another session.

The doctor began the conversation by asking if she had taken her medication, did she sleep better, and was she any less depressed. The agent told the doctor she had spoken to her husband on the phone the previous day and after the conversation she felt very depressed. The doctor asked if she had felt like calling him after her conversation with her husband. She told him she had just imagined talking to him. The doctor then changed the subject to a dream she had made reference to in a prior session wherein she remembered waking up and having a climax. The agent told the doctor about another dream which had nothing to do with sex. The doctor then brought the subject back to the sexual dream. He asked the agent if she would like her psychiatrist to be nice to her and if she wanted to please him. She stated she wanted him to think OK of her. He asked the agent why her husband wanted a divorce. She stated he feels she is a lousy wife, mother, and lover. She stated this was not true, she was good at all these things. The doctor asked if she liked oral sex and if her sex partners enjoyed it also. He also asked if any of her sex partners had ever stimulated her orally and, if so, could she have an orgasm this way. She advised she had, after which he made a comment relative to the fact she could have a climax orally but not with penetration. The doctor then stated, most men like oral sex and asked if she had not yet discovered that.

The doctor then changed the subject and asked the agent if she had gained any weight. She advised she had gained several pounds. He had her stand up and turn around so that he could look at her. He stated she had a nice figure. The agent sat down and picked up a book which was on the doctor's desk and advised she was nervous and he should have something in his office for people to hold on to. The doctor stated, it wasn't the book she needed to hold, but his hands instead. At that point the agent began repeating the doctor's statements because he was speaking very softly. The investigator could overhear the agent repeat that the doctor wanted her to sit on his lap. Also overheard was a statement by the agent that she could feel his penis moving. Also overheard was a statement by the agent that the doctor wanted her to kneel down in front of him. There were several minutes of unintelligible conversations after which I heard the agent say, "Why are you doing this to me?" At that point I left my vehicle and went into the office, identified myself and effected the arrest. The doctor resisted being placed in handcuffs, stating he was going to telephone his attorney before he went anywhere. The doctor was handcuffed and placed in the rear of my vehicle. At that time I advised him he was being arrested . . . and of his rights per the *Miranda* decision.

The state medical board forwarded to the county's district attorney the evidence it had collected against the psychiatrist, but the chief deputy district attorney felt there was "insufficient evidence to pursue filing charges." In his opinion, "the language of the statute prescribing conduct which is unprofessional or gross immorality is so big and uncertain that the law is probably defective." Although the investigators had compiled the testimony of former patients and a reconstruction (but not a tape recording) of the events that took place during the undercover operation, the vagueness of the statute, the doctor's subsequent strong denials of wrongdoing, and the legal difficulties of proving that the situation was not entrapment but attempted rape, all contributed to the prosecutor's reluctance to go forward.

Sexual Exploitation of the Sick.   Taped confrontations involving patients did help bring about the conviction of a psychiatrist on charges of Medi-Cal fraud and his subsequent dismissal from the program. The case was initiated when two female patients reported through a university professor that the doctor billed Medi-Cal for psychotherapy sessions that in fact consisted only of sexual activity with them. Both women had been diagnosed as manic-depressive, and both were said to be suicidal. One of the women first became a patient of the psychiatrist when she was hospitalized after an attempted suicide. She reported that he became romantic with her and allowed her to leave the hospital for a day, when he had intercourse with her at his home. He released her from the hospital about a week later. She then went to his office for treatment three times a week for the first month, and once a week thereafter. The doctor billed Medi-Cal for these visits, which, according to the patient, consisted almost entirely of sexual intercourse.

The patients helped the police by secretly taping meetings with the psychiatrist in which he acknowledged his sexual involvement with them. One of the patients asked him how he felt about getting paid to have sex with her. He told her he didn't feel very good about it. He said he regretted his behavior, was depressed at the time, and was looking for intimacy. He told her that sex with her "was an expression of our being close, of getting involved emotionally, and of my not making the boundaries clear."

This psychiatrist told another patient that "the next time she was making love to imagine it was him she was having sex with." He also had sexual intercourse with her during a camping trip. According to the investigative report:

He persuaded her to go camping when he told her that a friend of his, who was also a therapist, would also be with them along with some of his patients. He reassured her that "nothing would happen." He also told her, "You have nothing to worry about, chaperons will be around." The suspect picked her up in the evening. They then drove to pick up his friend and the others. While en route he unzipped his pants and took out his penis, and said, "I don't care about Bill or anyone else, I'm going to stick this thing in you tonight." He then took her hand and tried to hold it on his penis. She kept trying to pull her hand away, but he kept pulling it back on to his penis.

They met his friend Bill in a parking lot. But he was alone, saying the others couldn't make it. While Bill drove, the doctor again unzipped his pants and removed his penis. He took her hand and put it on his penis. She told him she didn't want to do this and kept pulling back. He told her that she "owed" it to him because Medi-Cal didn't pay him enough for his services treating her.

A few days after they returned from camping, he telephoned her before a group session. He told her to be "discreet" about the camping trip, especially around his wife, who would be at the group. That night after the group meeting, she went home and attempted suicide by taking more than forty lithium pills. She said she was feeling depressed and confused by the sexual relationship. Later he advised her how to commit suicide with lithium by taking smaller doses of ten pills at a time. She was scared that she would do it and thought she had to keep receiving treatment from him. He told her that he would keep her as a patient and that sometimes they would talk and sometimes they would have sex.

In this case, the MFCU filed criminal charges against the doctor for charging Medi-Cal for his liaisons. The district attorney declined to file sexual assault charges because "the sexual conduct was not the result of force in the usual sense." At the sentencing the defendant's attorney argued that the doctor had already been punished, suffering "public humiliation and other ancillary consequences of criminal acts." The prosecutor rebutted this view: "It is important to remember that the ancillary losses suffered by a white-collar criminal are of advantages not enjoyed by many other defendants coming before the court for sentencing. Neither the legislature nor the judicial counsel in enacting the rules of court suggested that the loss of professional privileges, public humiliation, and dissolution of marriage are factors to be considered in mitigation of punishment."

The court placed the psychiatrist on three years' probation, ordered him to pay $2,000 restitution, fined him a paltry $10, and ordered a six-month jail term and continuing psychiatric counseling. The state licensing board placed the psychiatrist on ten years' probation, which allowed the doctor to practice only in a supervised setting. One of the patients sued and settled for $200,000.

More Sex as Therapy.   Another psychiatrist prescribed large amounts of drugs for his wife, took drugs himself, treated patients while he was on drugs, and billed the government for psychotherapy during hours he spent having oral sex with the patient for whom he prescribed excessive drugs; he paid her $10 to $20 for each sex act.

Another case involved a "moonlighting" army psychiatrist who collected Medi-Cal payment stickers from several emotionally disturbed patients and for each of their children. He had repeatedly billed for full forty-five-minute individual psychotherapy sessions for each of the children without ever seeing them. By submitting false claims for sessions with five children and two women, he fraudulently obtained

$3,852. During the same period, he maintained a sexual relationship with a Medi-Cal recipient for which he billed the program $1,184 for forty-five-minute therapy sessions that were actually sexual and social encounters, many of which lasted only a few minutes. The patient reported that the doctor had taken her to various San Francisco hotels, had sexual relations with her, and demanded her Medi-Cal card in order to deceive his wife, who was also his bookkeeper.

An investigator for the California Board of Medical Quality Assurance discovered the psychiatrist's misconduct when a patient who had borne a child by him filed a lawsuit charging the doctor with child stealing after he took the baby and fled to Hawaii. These charges were dropped when he returned the baby and agreed to pay child support. The psychiatrist pled guilty to five counts of fraud, so all other counts against him were dismissed. He was ordered to serve one year in county jail and to pay $5,036 in restitution. He was also placed on probation for three years.

All these psychiatrists who conducted sexual liaisons with patients could have been prosecuted for Medicaid fraud, in addition to suffering regulatory sanctions. But in cases of sexual misconduct, patient abuse, rather than fraud, becomes the dominant issue for the authorities. The presiding judge in the last case commented on the absence of criminal charges against the psychiatrist:

I think that the Medi-Cal fraud was circumstantial evidence that didn't bear very heavily on it [the case]. I think the thing that the medical experts stated was the biggest violation of his standard of care to a patient was that of becoming personally involved with the patient under his care, which is strictly prohibited, particularly among psychiatrists, because of the nature of the illness they're treating; and second, yes, abuse of prescription rights would be seriously frowned on by the Medi-Cal people. They frown on both the improper treatment, the psychiatric treatment, and the proper medication. Medi-Cal fraud,. . . . honestly, was not so much an issue.

CONCLUSION

The judge's comments that Medicaid fraud may not be much of an issue with medical professionals may help explain the comparatively lenient punishment doctors receive. Abuse and exploitation of patients and of prescription-writing privileges disturb colleagues, but stealing money from benefit programs lacks, for both colleagues and judges, "the brimstone smell."[5] Without doctors' testimony condemning fraudulent conditions, judges are unlikely to mete out heavy sentences.

In sentencing physicians, the courts look beyond the offenses committed. As one federal judge explains:

I didn't want to send him to jail because I felt that it would deprive him and his family of the livelihood he could make as a doctor and it would deprive the neighborhood of his services. So what I was trying to accomplish was to see that to some extent he could repay society. In this particular case there was a strong enough reason to overcome whatever good would be done for society by imposing a sentence for general deterrence, which is the only justification that exists for [prison] sentences in these cases.[6]

The relative leniency expressed by judges and colleagues with respect to physician criminality most certainly contributes to the extent of the behaviors. Lacking censure, errant physicians practice without proper parameters of behavior. They are unlikely to perceive their own acts as criminal when others do not.

Chapter Five

Doctors Tell Their Stories

In the course of our research we interviewed forty-two physicians apprehended for Medicaid scams. To hear them tell it, they were innocent sacrificial lambs led to the slaughter because of perfidy, stupid laws, bureaucratic nonsense, and incompetent bookkeepers. At worst, they had been a bit careless in their record keeping; but mostly they had been more interested in the welfare of their patients than in deciphering the arcane requirements of benefit programs. Certainly, the Medicaid laws are complex and, by many reasonable standards, unreasonable. But we were surprised by the number of rationalizations that these doctors offered, by the intensity of their defenses of their misconduct, and by their consummate skill in identifying the villains who, out of malevolence or ineptitude, had caused their downfall. In these doctors' system of moral accounting, their humanitarian deeds far outweighed their petty trespasses against Medicaid.

THE RESEARCH APPROACH

Our task was a delicate one: to ask doctors to discuss their encounters with Medicaid enforcement officials. We presumed that we needed to appear as nonthreatening as possible without seeming to be so sympathetic or naive as to give credence to anything the respondents said. Walking this fine line required tact, patience, and at times a thick skin. Doctors are not accustomed to having what they say questioned; usually they are in firm control of situations involving their professional lives.

We wanted them to relive, in front of total strangers, what must have been some of the worst moments of their lives. Our goal was to find out as much as we could about why they behaved as they did, how and why they got caught, how their cases were handled, what punishments they received, how their experiences changed their attitudes and behavior, and how they would alter the Medicaid program to prevent situations such as the ones in which they were involved.

Before each interview, we reviewed the case file, but we used this material during the interview only to help a doctor recall details. We made no attempt to be confrontive about discrepancies between a doctor's account and the official records. Rather, we behaved as good listeners who wanted to know the doctor's side of the story. This approach seemed to work well. Most of the doctors appeared to offer information freely and candidly, and many assumed the role of "instructor," hoping to teach us what was wrong with the government programs. The vast majority were friendly and cooperative, and many said they were grateful that someone was studying the problem.

We combined for interview purposes doctors who had been administratively sanctioned and those who had been convicted of fraudulent activities. Our work had convinced us that how a case had been handled was not important. One physician might plead guilty to a single felony; another doctor, who had committed essentially the same offense at a different time and place, would avoid criminal action. We were not able to determine which cases truly deserved—in our judgment—criminal sanctions and which should have been treated administratively.

The doctors we interviewed practiced in New York and California, the states with the largest Medicaid programs. Sanctions were usually imposed for practices uniquely related to Medicaid, though in some instances the Medicaid aspect was part of a much larger violative episode—such as the case of the psychiatrist who sexually exploited his patient and billed Medicaid for their liaisons. The latter action merely aggravated the fundamental offense of "improper professional conduct," which would have been sufficient to have him sanctioned.

We obtained case file material for sixty-four physicians who had been proceeded against successfully. Thirty were from California; thirty-four were from New York. New York State's Medicaid Fraud Control Unit provided brief summaries of fourteen cases, and the state's Department of Social Services, which administers the Medicaid program, supplied twenty summaries. We also obtained the names but not the files of sixty-one doctors sanctioned for Medicaid abuse in California.

The Interview Sample

All told, we collected identifying information on 125 doctors who had been sanctioned for Medicaid violations in New York and California. We wrote each doctor asking for his or her help in our scholarly research project; we made it clear that we were not associated with Medicaid or with state or federal law enforcement authorities. We told the doctors that we were interested in learning more about their particular cases and in hearing their ideas about problems in government medical programs and what should be done about them. In closing, we assured them that we would treat them as confidential sources and not attribute any comments to them by name. We said we would try to reach them by telephone in about a week, and we enclosed a return postcard so they could indicate a convenient time for us to contact them.

Many of the addresses we had been given were no longer correct; about a third of our letters were returned undelivered. Telephone books, medical directories, licensing board rosters, and medical school alumni associations were of some help, but we were unable to contact 19 of the 125 doctors in our pool. Of the remaining doctors, 43 did not respond to the letter and were not willing to speak with us on the telephone. Another 17 doctors told us they would not grant us an interview. Three physicians said they still had ongoing cases—either an additional violation or an appeal—and their attorneys had advised them not to discuss their situation with outsiders. One physician in the pool had died.

Forty-two physicians did grant us interviews. About one-third of the interviews were conducted by telephone, either for the convenience of the doctor or because of distance. All but a few of the interviews were tape-recorded, always with the respondent's permission.

We compared the case files of the doctors we interviewed and those of 46 physicians we were unable to interview. Of the five criteria for comparison—sex, medical specialty, legal charge, sanction (administrative or criminal), and penalty—we found only two statistically significant differences. In the area of legal charges, theft and larceny constituted 31 percent of the charges against the interviewed doctors compared to 54 percent among those not interviewed. There were about the same number of false claim charges and drug- and sex-related allegations. The second difference concerned the punishments: Community service had been ordered for 23 percent of those who granted interviews, compared to only 11 percent of those to whom we did not speak.

Ninety-five percent of the offenders in each group were males. In both groups, about one-third were general practitioners; about a third of those interviewed and a quarter of those not interviewed were psychiatrists. The charges against the doctors were essentially similar for both groups, and about two-thirds of the violators in both had been convicted of crimes. The overall similarity between the two groups strongly suggests that the doctors we interviewed were reasonably representative of sanctioned physician Medicaid violators from the two jurisdictions we studied.

The Control Group

Our intention was to employ a "quasi-matched control group design" that would enable us to compare the responses of sanctioned physicians with a control group of Medicaid providers who had not been sanctioned for fraud or abuse. The absence of official rosters of Medicaid providers categorized by such characteristics as age, specialty, and location frustrated this aim, but we were able to put together a control group that did not appear to vary in significant ways from the characteristics of the sanctioned interviewees.

Because 79 percent of our face-to-face interviews were conducted in California, mainly Southern California, we selected members of our comparison group from that area. We consulted the classified telephone directories for Los Angeles County and called the physicians listed as being in "General Practice"; we asked their receptionists (or, in a few instances, the doctors) whether the doctors accepted Medi-Cal patients.

Those who did were sent a cover letter, along with a return postcard, requesting an interview. We automatically sent a letter to general practitioners and specialists who specifically stated in their advertisements that they took Medi-Cal patients. Predictably, the sample for a city such as Los Angeles was heavily weighted toward areas predominantly occupied by members of minority groups (East Los Angeles, Culver City, Inglewood, and Hawthorne).

To ensure that we would make contact with a sufficient number of psychiatrists, we obtained from the Los Angeles County Medical Association the names of some of those who accepted Medi-Cal. Association policy is to respond to a telephone inquiry by providing a random selection of the names of three doctors in a specified community. We simply made repeated telephone calls to the bemused receptionist in order to generate our list, focusing on communities likely to have a large number of patients who use Medi-Cal. These procedures provided a remarkably well-matched group of physicians—at least on the dimensions we were able to measure.

The response rate from our letters and calls was much lower in the control group: Only 16 percent (32 of 212 physicians) agreed to be interviewed, compared to the 40 percent response rate from the sanctioned doctors. We were unable to determine whether the nonsanctioned physicians were less interested in the topic of our study or whether they were just too busy. (Many of the sanctioned doctors told us they now had time on their hands, since their practices had declined after the government actions against them.)

We found no statistically significant differences between the sanctioned and nonsanctioned doctors in regard to where they had been trained: About 70 percent of each group were educated in American schools of medicine or osteopathy. Thirty-six percent of the sanctioned group and 29 percent of the comparison group had attended the same university for both their undergraduate education and their medical training, a difference not statistically significant.

Marital status and ethnicity were essentially similar for both groups, as was the predominance of solo practitioners (76 percent of the sanctioned group and 65 percent of the comparison cohort). About 70 percent of each group reported no other business interests beyond their medical practice, and most physicians in each group reported having a variety of friends rather than having social associations only with business or professional colleagues.

Members of the sanctioned group, however, were significantly older than the comparison doctors—a finding that we believe is relevant to understanding the motives of the violators. The average age of the sanctioned doctors was 57.2 years, compared to 48.2 for the nonsanctioned group. The groups also differed in the number of locations in which they had practiced: an average of 2.6 sites for the sanctioned group and 1.9 for the control group, another statistically significant difference. We could not discern, however, whether this difference reflected some instability in the careers of the sanctioned doctors; whether it indicated upward, downward, or lateral mobility; or whether it was merely an artifact of their longer periods of practice.

RATIONALES AND RATIONALIZATIONS

The sanctioned doctors generally appeared open and candid, at ease and involved with the subject. Most were perfectly accurate in response to our opening question—which asked them to provide the factual details of their cases—though these recitals were interladen with a plethora of self-excusatory observations. Throughout the interview, we gave the respondents a great deal of leeway in responding, and we sought to avoid putting words in their mouths or guiding them in any particular direction. They could be rude or polite to us (most were very polite), satisfied or disgusted with the government, and optimistic or pessimistic about the futures of their careers. At times, some doctors told us more than they realized. It is difficult in a long, sometimes emotional interview to camouflage strongly held convictions.

All the doctors in the sanctioned group had been suspended from billing the Medicaid program, and about two-thirds had been convicted of a criminal offense. Nonetheless, a doctor often would ask us, "What did I do that was so bad?" Clearly, their interpretations of the ethical and legal character of their actions were quite unlike those made by the law enforcement authorities.

One way to explain this dissonance is by reference to the classic sociological work of Gresham Sykes and David Matza on juvenile delinquents. According to Sykes and Matza, these young criminals "neutralize" the negative definitions that they know "respectable" people apply to their delinquent behaviors. By learning these neutralization techniques in delinquent subcultures, juveniles can render social controls inoperative and be free to engage in delinquency without serious harm to their self-images. Thus, the delinquent can remain committed to law-abiding norms but can also "qualify" them in order to make violations excusable, if not altogether "right." Sykes and Matza observe that "much delinquency is based on what is essentially an unrecognized extension of defenses to crimes, in the form of justifications for deviance that are seen as valid by the delinquent but not by the legal system or society at large."[1] From a study of embezzlers incarcerated in federal prisons, Donald Cressey concluded that these wrongdoers used "vocabularies of adjustment" to justify their behaviors to themselves. They told themselves that they were merely "borrowing" the money, which they would replace just as soon as they resolved a momentary problem. This self-deception enabled the embezzlers to see themselves as basically decent although they were altering records and stealing money.[2]

Because we carried out our interviews several years after the offenses had taken place, we could not determine whether the doctors had fashioned their explanations before or after they committed the abuses—an analytical issue that has bedeviled all researchers attempting to verify the importance of neutralization techniques in lawbreaking. Most likely, we heard explanations of both types. Our data do tend to support the hypothesis that neutralization often constitutes an important element of what has been called the "drift" into illegal behavior, a period during which the perpetrator's episodic lawbreaking often goes unattended and thus begins to lose whatever unsavory moral flavor it might have possessed.[3]

Denial of Responsibility

Few physicians took full personal blame for their violations in the sense of describing them as volitional, deliberate acts of wrongdoing. They were apt to call their activities "mistakes," and some blamed themselves for not having been more careful. This neutralization practice corresponds to what Sykes and Matza call denial of responsibility: "Denial of responsibility . . . extends much further than the claim that deviant acts are an 'accident' or some similar negation of personal accountability. . . . By learning to view himself as more acted upon than acting, the delinquent prepares the way for deviance from the normative system without the necessity of a frontal assault on the norms themselves."[4]

The wrongdoing physicians did engage in a frontal assault on Medicaid norms, but they typically laid the blame on a wide variety of persons other than themselves. Several blamed patients' demands, portraying their own behavior as altruistic. One insisted she was doing no more than trying to see to the essential health of needy people: "Some of the kids didn't have any Medicaid, and you get a mother saying, 'Look, my child is sick. I don't have any Medicaid. Could you put it on the other kid's Medicaid?' It probably wasn't their child to begin with. It was like a sister's child." The physician admitted that she complied with the mother's request, and her "goodheartedness" got her into trouble with the government. She says that during the investigation, "the mother who brought in her sister's child forgot that this kid was treated because it was like a year ago." The mother's lapse of memory or fabrication, the doctor suspected, occurred because the mother hoped to avoid implicating herself in the fraud.

The same physician also insisted she had been victimized by thieves who stole Medicaid cards from beneficiaries and then presented themselves for treatment. Her practice was in "a bad area," and such thefts were common, she pointed out. When the itemization of treatment services came to the legitimate cardholders, they would complain to the authorities. Even if this was true, however, her explanation sidestepped the issue of her responsibility to match the Medicaid card with the person presenting it.

A psychiatrist also argued that his problems resulted from the irresponsibility of a patient, a young woman with whom he had had sexual relations. He had charged Medi-Cal for the time he spent with his mistress only so that his wife, who handled some of his billing, would not become suspicious:

People knew I was seeing this individual after-hours, when the staff went home. My wife knew I was down at the office. So the only way to cover that visit and not let there be any suspicion was to bill Medi-Cal. The purpose was not to defraud Medi-Cal in the pure sense of making money. It was to simply protect the relationship, so my wife wouldn't be suspicious. Why am I seeing a person and not charging them anything? She [the mistress] was totally in agreement. I mean, it was the only basis on which we would be allowed to continue. It was her suggestion. "Why don't you just continue to put in the charges under Medi-Cal? I am not going to blow the whistle on you." So she was in the scheme as well as I was.

He portrayed the woman as the initiator and aggressor in the affair:

She came back to the office . . . to see whether I was still friendly to her or what the relationship would be, and so she came in as though she were a patient. I mean my office staff made an appointment for her, and what have you, and then she contacted me on the phone later and asked if I would be willing to continue seeing her. I said "fine" to satisfy mutual desires, so to speak, and we continued to see each other about a dozen times within six to eight months.

The doctor was well aware that he was in a hazardous situation; indeed, he explained in some detail why he should not have done what he did:

There is a rule of thumb, at least in the area of psychiatry and psychology, not so much in general medical practice, and that is that you don't become personally involved with your patients. But that is not common among doctors. That is, most doctors at some time or another do get involved with patients. But you shouldn't do it in psychology and psychiatry because you get too involved personally, and you really have to maintain a distance. Otherwise you cannot be effective. Or else if you get involved, you should definitely make sure that some other colleague is seeing the patient and working with him, if they still need help, and not be dependent on yourself, because you can't be objective. One thing you don't do is, you know, really try to be a psychiatrist to your own lover or wife, or whatever. That's really poor judgment.

By blaming the patient for initiating the sexual relationship and the Medi-Cal fraud, the psychiatrist was able to neutralize his guilt about violating ethical and legal standards. He further buttressed his self-image as an altruistic human being by suggesting that he was doing his mistress-patient a favor, in view of how demanding his practice was:

I carried a very, very heavy load. So it really was very difficult for me to. . . . There were only a couple of occasions in the whole time I was able to literally squeeze in a visit—on a couple of occasions to her apartment on the way home from the hospital. But it was very hard to arrange those things. . . . One time when I was in the apartment, it really almost got me trapped. I got a beeper call while I was at her apartment. I was really flustered about the whole thing. I realized that I really didn't have the time or freedom at all. So it kind of put a damper on that. It was very difficult.

We then asked the psychiatrist whether, in order to conceal the relationship from his wife, he would have accepted a fee from the patient if she were paying it out of her own pocket. In a barrage of confused verbiage, he sought to reestablish a satisfying neutralization to exculpate himself:

Yeah, if she had private insurance. Well, it would have been difficult to even do that. But possibly if it would have been a private insurance or if it would have been something that she would have to pay out of her pocket, I might have tried some way to personally reimburse her. You know what I'm saying? But if that is something she wanted or felt was only right to do. Obviously, I couldn't reimburse the government without making it obvious. But there would have been a way to do that.

Now there would have to be a way to do insurance if she was covered with insurance. It was to either work some kind of a scheme out there. But if it was personal, and I assume if our relationship was good enough, I would have probably said to her, "I could find out a way to get cash, you know, sufficient cash and get it back to you, if you feel that." See, the only condition under which I was willing to continue to see her was that we had to cover ourselves as far as our visits were concerned, and in most cases the visits were in the office, and the only way I could cover it was either to bill her—I would have had to bill her. If she had to pay and was billed and said, "I don't want to pay," and obviously I wasn't going to pay her back. So the whole purpose of the deceit to Medi-Cal, I believe, was exactly the way it would have been if it were private—to not let anybody become suspicious, and there would have been no way for them not to become suspicious if they weren't billed. I feel this way, there would have been no reason not to have exactly the same procedure knowing that she was better off, because the point was not the money. It was the deception.

Ultimately, the patient brought a malpractice suit against the psychiatrist. In his closing argument the doctor's attorney compared the plaintiff to a prostitute. Her attorney countered tellingly: "A prostitute is one who receives money for sex. There is only one person in the room that I know of who did that."

Patients were not the only individuals physicians blamed for their troubles with the law. Business managers and employees were commonly designated as the true culprits. One psychiatrist, who billed the government for hour-long therapy sessions that were actually much shorter, blamed a new billing clerk, though he granted that his supervision might have been better:

I got a big formidable black girl who said she had worked for Medicaid/Medicare in Washington, D.C. One of the doctors in town had a wife, a nurse, who called and said there was this wonderful girl. "I know you're having trouble collecting. She did wonders for us." And I said, "I'll take her and just give her a dollar an hour more than you did." We went from collecting nothing to six, seven thousand dollars a month from Medi-Cal and Medicare, and another 10 or 15 percent from other insurance.

I used to ask her, "Geez, where's the money coming from? Are you sure we're not doing something wrong?" And her answer was, "No, you're a specialist. You're accepting the rates for nonspecialized men. You're highly specialized. You've been doing this for twenty-five years."

The non sequitur here, of course, is that his being a specialist could not have borne any relationship to his sudden ability to collect thousands of dollars each month when, as he tells it, he had been "having trouble collecting" and getting "nothing" each month.

The psychiatrist continued his tale of the wayward clerk with the following version of how she got him into such trouble:

She was a smart kid. She was twenty-four, had two children of her own, was divorced from a military officer, and had a brother with her. A real strong black woman. So, as it turned out later on, she was keeping books for other doctors around town, and nothing happened to her.

She wasn't making any money with our stealing and fraud. She had it so well organized that I suppose I might have resented her coming in an hour for two days per week instead of the original thirty hours that we might have agreed on. But it was running so damn well, who'd complain?

I read in the *L.A. Times* about a psychologist who had billed for 160 hours in one week. Well, there are only 168 hours, see. I took it out and stuck it on the wall by the girl's big desk over there. I asked her, "We wouldn't be doing something like that, would we?" I kind of had a laugh. I thought: "Does that kid know there are only 168 hours in one week?" I asked her: "I'm getting all this goddamned money. Are you sure this is the way it should be coming in? There aren't that many hours in a week."

Another physician got into trouble for accepting kickbacks from a laboratory. (Physicians can bill Medicaid for laboratory tests if they own the testing facility; otherwise the laboratory bills Medicaid.) This physician told us he had decided to do his own lab work in order to increase his income. A former employee, whom the physician held responsible for his misfortune, offered the doctor a deal:

My lab technician quit to start his own laboratory. He said: "Why don't you give me all the lab work." I said: "Fine, you bill Medicaid, and I'll bill my private patients."

They were doing the tests for so much, and I charged them the going rate, and he was giving me a good deal, and that was a private deal. The Medi-Cal, he was doing it all and billing it himself.

Then I told him: "I'm going to get a technician so I can have the benefits of the laboratory, of Medi-Cal too." [But] eventually he says: "I'll give you some benefits on your private patients. For instance, your bill is $300. I'll cut it down to $200 or something so we'll make it up somehow." I said: "All right."

Another physician who took kickbacks portrayed himself as an unwary, passive participant, motivated only by amiability and generosity, in a plan hatched by a hospital. The initiative came from the hospital, and the direct beneficiaries were his employees, so, as far as he was concerned, he had done nothing wrong in allowing the hospital to underwrite his payroll:

Hospital, privately owned, was in the habit of giving kickbacks to physicians using the hospital. I had arranged for three of the girls that worked for me to receive part-time pay to the tune of about $250 each, per month.

This lasted about two years before it was stopped, and the amount of work that they did for the money they received was negligible. So they were able to show in court that this was an indirect type of kickback. Even though the money was not paid to me, by the girls receiving this money, it obviously made them happier or better employees or whatever you want to call it.

I felt that if I didn't accept it, that if I let the girls take it, and then made sure that they got their full salaries and their Christmas bonuses, that I wasn't actually getting any benefit out of it. I thought that therefore I was immune.

And I really wasn't getting any benefit out of it. I had three employees—two of them were getting divorces, and one of them had a third child. The hospital wanted to give kickbacks, let them have it, you know.

An obstetrician, perhaps truthfully, cast responsibility on the welfare department, which had told him how to circumvent an inconvenient regulation:

Even the [welfare] department told me to change dates . . . to be within the letter of the law. For example, some girl delivers the baby, she decides to have her tubes tied. Now, according to the state, there has to be an application thirty days ahead of tubular ligation, and it has to be submitted, approved, and thirty days given for the patient to make up her mind, to decide.

If she hadn't given us any indication to the ligation, and she has to have one, what do we do now? I can't say, "You have to go home and come back in thirty days." And so they [the welfare caseworkers] told me, as well as the other doctors for Medicaid, they'd just say: "Backdate the request thirty days."

Commonly, denials of responsibility were blended with other self-justifications. A psychiatrist who illegally submitted bills under his name (and took a cut) for work done by psychologists not qualified for payment under Medicaid blamed the therapists but also added that he did it for the benefit of his patients:

There were times I wanted to quit, but the therapist would say that these people are in need of therapy, and it is going along well. It seemed to make sense at the time. They were qualified people. I couldn't do it myself; I wasn't there all the time. It was partly a moral thing. I was persuaded to keep doing it, and a good percentage of patients were getting something out of it. I should have been more responsible, but it also had to do with my trust in people, and that trust was misplaced.

This physician, perhaps as a reflexive bow to a major postulate of his vocation, commented, "I don't want to think of myself as a victim, so I want to take responsibility for what I did." Yet he found irresistible the idea that it was his essential goodness—his trust in people and his sympathy for patients—that had led him astray.

Denial of Injury

Justifying lawbreaking by citing the superordinate benefits of the act—such as the psychiatrist's comment on the value of the therapy for his patients—is called denial of injury in the roster of Sykes and Matza's techniques of neutralization. As they point out, "wrongfulness may turn on the question of whether or not anyone has clearly been hurt by [the] deviance, and this matter is open to a variety of interpretations."[5] Physicians often depicted Medicaid regulations, which assuredly can be both onerous and mercilessly nitpicking, as bureaucratic obstacles, erected by laypeople, that threatened patient care. By breaking or bending the Medicaid rules, the sanctioned physicians argued, they were responding to their higher calling and helping—not hurting— patients.

Taking this tack, a physician who treated obesity by performing surgery emphasized that he was motivated only by "medical reasons" and "didn't give a goddamn what Medi-Cal said":

Consider patients on welfare. There's a huge group of people who are on welfare because they cannot work. Nobody will give them a job. Their obesity serves as an excuse for remaining in the welfare system. To themselves they just say: "Well, I'm fat; I cannot get a job; therefore, I have to be on welfare." And they're satisfied with it. To alter that situation is hazardous, both from the emotional standpoint, but particularly in terms of physical aspects of it because if they eat enough, no matter how you loused up their gut, they're going to manage to remain obese. Earlier on, fifteen years ago, I did a few welfare patients, and I soon recognized the problem that particular group has espe- cially. The bottom line is that there is a subconscious need for obesity.

Well, I came up with the idea many years ago of saying: "OK, if you want this done, I've got no handle on what your subconscious state is, how much you need your obesity; there's no test for it. But the pocketbook is pretty close to the subconscious mind. If you are willing to pay for something, chances are you want it." Doesn't work that great; but at least it's a way. So what I started doing was charging them in advance: You want surgery, you come up with the money. Your insurance company happens to pay it back, you know, pay the full fee; well, I'll give it right back to them.

I must admit that I did some Medi-Cal patients before I came up with this gimmick. And one or two of them worked very well. They became employable and very successful. But on the other hand, for every successful one, I would find two or three that became a disaster and had to be taken down and reoperated, all kinds of problems.

So, anyway, I started this business. So I go: "OK, you want this surgery; you pay half of it." Now, at that particular point in time, I didn't give a goddamn what Medi-Cal said. I mean, if the patient wants this done, whether it's legal or illegal. I said I'm doing this for my reasons—medical reasons. What they'd have to come up with was maybe $100 or $500, whatever. The fee that Medi-Cal was paying at that time, plus the $500, was still less than what it would be for a private patient. Medi-Cal was paying maybe $500 or $600.

I didn't give a damn about the money. It wasn't as if I got a patient in the emergency room and Medi-Cal only paid me $150, but my fee was $600, and so I tried to collect the balance. That wasn't my intent at all. Welfare patients do not expect to pay you. But this was a volitional thing. They knew about it in advance. It was not an emergency. It was purely elective, cosmetic. I knew I couldn't bill. That's the only part of the regulations I knew and recognized.

It wasn't as though there was fraud involved. I wasn't defrauding anybody. If you want this surgery, you pay me before surgery, not afterwards. If I were billing them afterwards, I recognize that was bad. But this isn't the same thing. I still don't think so.

I really thought I had some really nice results on a few of them. I did have some disasters. That is why I started this. If I had just had the disasters and said "the hell with it, there's no answer to this, get out," I would have avoided it, because I didn't need it. It didn't amount to that much money. I could have been doing a private patient and come out way ahead.

Of course, the physician could have employed tactics other than reaching into a beneficiary's wallet to determine the patient's motivation—for example, adherence to a diet and exercise regimen prior to the operation. That the preoperative payment was intended to preclude reneging on the fee, rather than to measure motivation, is implicit in the physician's subsequent statement:

Now, plastic surgeons, for example, have done this for years. If you want to have your nose fixed, you pay them right up front. And for the same reason. Because they know that if you have to try to collect afterwards, the patient's going to find five hundred reasons why their nose isn't the way they thought it was going to be. If you've already paid for it, they'll be happy and satisfied.

Such comparisons with other specialties were common among doctors seeking to explain away their violations of the law. The Medicaid rules were capricious, and their own interpretation of fairness was far more sensible than that of the bureaucrats. Consider this psychiatrist's self-righteous indignation:

My wife is an eminently qualified psychiatric nurse. She had a medical teaching appointment on a medical school staff, supervisor of their inpatients, very qualified individual. So, anyhow, the basic problem was, she worked for me. They accused me—I don't know what the hell they accused me of—charging [Medicaid] for her services.

She was my nurse employee, just like I've had nurse employees everywhere I've been. I have always billed, like when the nurse gave a shot, you didn't bill it through her name. I don't even understand this concept, you know. I still don't understand what basis they can say arbitrarily that she is any different than a nurse that works for an obstetrician.

The way people are supervised in psychiatry is different than for general medicine. They never understood the difference, and still don't, and don't want to know. You can't talk with other physicians about it because they don't know anything about psychiatry, and don't want to know. You are in an esoteric field, that you have to be in to understand.

In a similar vein, another psychiatrist found the regulations senseless and the work he was doing eminently valuable for his patients. Besides, he had been able to bill in another setting for therapy provided by nonphysicians, so he could not comprehend why such an action was not permitted under Medi-Cal:

I worked as a convalescent lead psychiatrist at one time. Now that means working in one of these county clinics where you are seeing patients and the social worker is seeing patients. These people are being charged the full rate, and it is only the psychiatrist who has a Medi-Cal number. If it is all right in the agency, why isn't it all right in private practice?

I was aware of putting down my name and not any other therapist, you know, who wouldn't be honored. But nevertheless, they were still my patients, and everything that went on was under my signature and my supervision. Some social workers are better than some psychiatrists in the analysis of a problem. Some psychiatrists are not that good in understanding human behavior.

I will stand by unequivocally that the patients that were seen by me, in conjunction with others, were getting far more for their dollar, whether it is paid for by them, their company, or by Medi-Cal. They were getting far more from my clinic than they would get anywhere from one practitioner, and it was because there were certain areas in my training and intuition, my skills, where someone else could do better, and vice versa. As far as I am concerned, they are quality people—something I insisted upon.

My idea was with Medi-Cal, or with whatever I was doing, do what was right for the patients and for the patients' good. I consider four eyes better than two eyes, four arms better than two arms, and four ears better than two ears, and these patients were getting more in their hourly fee.

As noted earlier, the mean age of the sanctioned doctors was nine years above that of the nonsanctioned comparison group. Presumably, the older practitioners had entered medical practice before Medicaid had been established, and some may have been unwilling to change their ways to conform to Medicaid's rules. For example, some older doctors may not stay fully abreast of current medical developments and may persist in idiosyncratic treatment methods. No one within the profession is likely to challenge them, but Medicaid will deny payment for "unacceptable" procedures.

Consider the case of an elderly physician who prescribed large doses of Ritalin, an amphetamine, to treat alcoholism. Ritalin is approved for medical use only when the diagnosis is hyperactivity in a child or narcolepsy in an adult:

There were a few patients who tended to drift over to my office, and these patients were people who had apparently had wide treatment for alcoholism with Ritalin. I decided I would try this on a limited basis. For all my practicing years, I had never found anything that was really effective with the treatment of alcoholism. So I put two patients of mine on Ritalin. The treatment seemed to make sense to me. I treated them for a month or so, and I found other people trickling into my office and then a flood. And this continued for a year.

Ritalin is a drug used on aberrant children with autistic tendencies. And it's used in doses that are remarkably like those that I was using in the treatment of alcoholism, so I didn't feel out of order. I prescribed 20 milligrams, three times a day.

If Ritalin has any effect over alcoholism, I think it is a worthy drug to be using in my treatment. Alcohol is a severe depressant, and when one is depressed, he is robbed of the ability to think because he is always winding down, and nothing matters at the moment, so he can't think.

If Ritalin picked him up to a point where he could think, then he could suppress his alcoholism and increase his chances of living a temporarily active life as long as he took the Ritalin. Now Ritalin's effectiveness for alcoholism has never been proved one way or the other.

I look at medicine as being a practice where the overall good of the practice, whatever it may be, should be the primary guiding factor. In other words, if you have one person die of the use of Ritalin, and if you have thousands of persons die with alcoholism, where is the sense of that?

Despite this doctor's assertion that "the treatment seemed to make sense," Ritalin is a tightly controlled substance, and his behavior was a serious offense. Moreover, the dosages he prescribed—20 milligrams three times a day—were excessive and probably resulted in his patients' reselling the drug on the street.

Another physician in his seventies got into trouble for failing to keep adequate records. In his patients' files he would note a prescription, but little else—a serious violation. The doctor explained his disagreement with the government this way: "They felt that I had not documented sufficiently the patients' records. I don't think so. I recorded notes each time the patients visited. Then I would record the medications prescribed. There is no need to write volumes because records are solely for my own purposes." To his way of thinking, the records were his private papers, not documents that might be needed by other doctors to ensure continuity of care.

One elderly practitioner took the government investigators to task over the definition of "good faith": "Their claim was that I was prescribing drugs without a good faith physical examination. However, what constitutes 'good faith' is a question, because the medical examination that the law requires does not mean a physical. Seeing the patients in the office constitutes a medical examination. You talk to patients; that's a medical examination." More recent medical school graduates, however, probably would assume that the medical examination required before prescribing a drug would involve more than merely talking to the patient. Though the doctor's semantic dodge seemed to satisfy him, this justification wholly ignored the harm his casual approach might have inflicted on patients.

Another physician offered a summary statement supporting professional autonomy and dismissing unwarranted and undesirable bureaucratic intervention:

They [the Medicaid officials] are the ones who eventually look over all this and say: "No, that was wrong." Now their idea of right and wrong is very different from what is considered right and wrong by normal people, or by physicians who are not necessarily normal, but at least [have their own] ideas about what is right and wrong. And to us, right and wrong have to do with things like patient care, whether we give them the right treatments. It doesn't have anything to do with some Medicaid regulation.

Denial of a Victim

A third neutralization technique, denial of a victim, occurs when an offender grants that his or her behavior caused injury but insists "the injury is not wrong in light of the circumstances."[6] In our interviews, the sanctioned physicians claimed that although the law had been broken, the excess reimbursement they had received represented only what they deserved for their work. They saw overcharging for services and ordering excessive tests as ways to "make back" what they *should* have been paid.

One physician, for example, granted that his excessive billings were wrong, especially because Medicaid participation was voluntary; but he maintained that the regulations and payment schedules encouraged— even necessitated—cheating, so that doctors in the program could earn fees equivalent to those paid by private insurance:

If you voluntarily choose to accept Medicaid patients, you have to put up with their baloney, and if you're not willing to put up with their baloney, then maybe you shouldn't take Medicaid patients. So in that sense, it's difficult to say something is not fair and you shouldn't do it. . . .

But the system has got many flaws in it and loopholes and irregularities which necessitate abuses to take place. Otherwise, you can't see patients because of the reimbursement attitude.

Let's take an example. A patient comes in for the first time and is examined. For that it would be, let's say, $60. Now, if the patient goes to a general practitioner for the first time with a cold, he [the doctor] will get that amount. If the patient goes to an internist, who has to evaluate the patient for a complicated situation, such as diabetes, heart disease, god knows what, and spends a lot of time with that patient, he will get compensated the same amount. So it's all the same because it is a new patient visit.

Now for that reason, it is virtually impossible to [receive treatment] at this time in this area. There are virtually no internists in this area that I know who accept Medicaid, because if a patient comes to an internist, they expect a thorough going-over, which they devote anywhere from half an hour to forty-five minutes, and yet the reimbursement rate is exactly the same as if the patient went to a general practitioner with a cold and spent five minutes with him.

Now the system, of course, does ask, when you bill for this visit, whether you spent a lot of time with the patient or a little time. You are supposed to voluntarily say that it was a brief visit and, if you state that, they will pay you a less amount. However, very few people I know do that. They will always bill the maximum amount because that maximum amount is actually less than we charge our private patients. This is one door of abuse that virtually everyone I know who takes Medicaid is using. If they billed the patient with a cold for a very brief visit, then they get paid as little as $12. There's no one I know who can function in this area, with an office and a staff and insurance and all these things, and accept a patient for $12. I would say that form of abuse exists in 90 to 100 percent of doctors that I know who take Medicaid. They're all using the maximum [reimbursement] levels.

This physician's conviction that virtually all his colleagues engaged in billing scams provided fuel for self-justification. As Sykes and Matza note, such a belief allows the perpetrator to transform the violation from "a gesture of complete opposition" to one that represents no more than "an extension of common practice."[7]

An anesthesiologist, caught billing the government for excess time, argued that he was reasonably charging for the patients' recovery time— a charge he knew was against Medicaid regulations:

We saw no reason why we should do abortions on the garbage of the ghettos and barrios and be responsible for their recovery time and not be paid for it. I really think that it was gray, not black. I'm not defending it. In the context of the time, it wasn't really that bad. But it was stupid to try and do it considering how little money was involved and the horrible consequences. I should have known better. If you are going to steal from the system, it was a very stupid act. I don't think it was really a basically crooked act. I guess you could say it was, but it depends on how you look at it.

When I did it, it was being done by at least 50 percent or 70 percent of the anesthesiologists in Southern California—at least 50 percent. People were fudging time, particularly on Medicaid.

Another physician also blamed the government for creating intolerable conditions that pressed practitioners toward fraud in order to meet patients' needs. The doctor illustrated what he saw as his dilemma by telling of a fourteen-year-old girl who was having her third abortion in less than six months. He had given the girl birth control pills, but she obviously hadn't taken them. When she came back for the third abortion, he coaxed her into allowing him to insert an IUD: "It's very simple, very easy. We'll put it in right now, immediately after the abortion."

The doctor then billed Medicaid for the IUD and its insertion, but the program would not pay because the insertion was done at the same time as the abortion for a fee the agency decreed reasonably covered both procedures. The doctor was irritated:

So they don't give a damn. It has to be a separate visit. So, then there's the question of getting this patient back. She's already got a local anesthetic in for the abortion. She says, "OK, do it. I won't feel it." You try to convince that same girl a week later or two weeks later? "Oh, no, I don't want those shots again" or "No, it's going to hurt. I don't want an IUD. I'll take the pill." It's another way of driving up costs. It drives up costs because they're going to have the girl pregnant again, and they're going to be perfectly willing to pay for more abortions rather than violate their rule. I paid $7, $8, $9 for an IUD. If I've been foolish enough to insert it immediately after an abortion—I can just forget getting paid. That's too bad. That's my problem. I should have made her come back in two weeks.

Now that's a medical decision that they have no business getting involved in. One of the ways I can handle this problem with this fourteen-year-old, if I've decided that the most important thing is her welfare, is I'm going to put in the goddamn IUD and put on the chart that I put it in tomorrow. Right? Because your health really should come before some bureaucrat, and there's no reason why I should be asked to throw away my money.

Another physician had essentially the same lament, one that also included an assessment of the kinds of people who receive Medicaid:

They say you cannot bill for more than one service rendered on one day. They forget what kind of patients the Medicaid patients are. They don't keep appointments. They don't keep regular checkups. I know that. And being conscientious, when a patient came with a problem, or I saw that it was three years that they had not yet come in, and they were coming in because they had a vaginal itch, I would treat for the vaginitis which prompted that visit, but also I performed the yearly checkup—Pap smear, breast examination, all that— urinalysis, et cetera—complete physical.

I knew that if I wanted to be within the strict letter of the law, I had to tell them to come tomorrow for the extra things—knowing that they would never come. They were poor. They didn't have transportation. So I used my better judgment and did everything they needed then. And to be within the program, I used next day's date, and that's where the problem was.

Various complaints about the nature of Medicaid recipients were offered by physicians in support of their view that Medicaid practice was more demanding than "normal" medicine and, by implication, should pay more rather than less. One doctor flaunted his disgust to us: "The Medicaid patients are filthy. They keep the place in turmoil. They are the toughest type to treat. The Medicaid patient is more demanding as a rule, and is not as cooperative in their treatment programs. I found this to be very troublesome at times."

Even if one were to accept the doctors' premise that the regulations were too inflexible given the difficulties of working with Medicaid patients, one has to wonder about the structural conflict between the physicians' interest in their patients' well-being and their own financial

self-interest. For example, the physician who inserted IUDs after performing abortions argued that he was offering important care to patients.
Yet he was unwilling to assume the small cost of the IUD and the
minimal extra time to insert it; instead, he chose to cheat Medicaid and
reap illegitimate profits. Before the advent of Medicaid, of course, many
physicians performed services for indigent patients without charge.
They spread the cost of care for the indigent among their fee-paying and
insured patients. Government benefit programs now offer—if one is
willing to cheat—the opportunity both to proclaim a humanitarian
interest in the welfare of poor patients and to get paid at or above the
going rate for that interest.

One physician we spoke with harkened to the theme of pro bono
service, but quickly added that he was always ready to circumvent the
law in order to obtain his fee from Medicaid:

> I would say personally I am disappointed with my colleagues in medicine. All
> of them are interested in their business. They are not concerned about the
> health of their patients. They want to make money. And, of course, they will
> make money. But the primary objective should be the care of patients. In
> medicine, the fee you get is a side effect.
>
> I was satisfied with the Medicaid reimbursement because I always knew that
> if somebody didn't pay me, my conscience would make me treat them anyway.
> I figured it was better to get Medicaid than to treat them free. Some of the
> regulations are annoying, but you could always get around them. I would first
> treat the patient, then deal with Medicaid.

This blend of decency, self-righteousness, and a thoroughly high-
handed attitude about "annoying" regulations that "you could always
get around" nicely satisfied this doctor's conscience and cash flow.

Getting around the rules, playing the Medicaid game, working the
system for maximum profit—many of the doctors we spoke with defined
their illegal activities in such terms. As one doctor observed:

> The ones that use the system play it, just like a musician plays an organ, you
> know. You play it to get the maximum response out of it. You know which
> buttons to push in order to get the kind of response that you want. . . . I've
> always looked upon it as a game; you're dealing with this big nebulous mon-
> strosity called the health care administration. The game was trying to extract

the maximal amount of money out of them to see if you could raise it up to the level that you get from others. . . . I would get absolutely no satisfaction in following the regulations to the letter, which give you very low reimbursement.

Let me put it this way. If after three years [of being suspended from the program], I regain the Medicaid status, I would probably not practice Medicaid. Because if you follow their regulations, reimbursement is so low that you could not maintain the old way with it. So in order to make a profit from it, you have to cheat almost. And I am certainly not in a position to do the slightest amount of cheating.

"Cheat almost" is a curious circumlocution that both minimizes the offenses and implies that doctors who do not cheat are running their practices at a financial loss. This physician, apparently, had come to believe that he was entitled to the highest income his practice could conceivably generate, even if that meant repeatedly breaking the law.

The same doctor offered a self-serving distinction between serious violations and "minor scams," which he thought were commonplace because the financial incentives were so irresistible:

I don't know anybody who is involved in major scams. I wasn't, and I don't have any sympathy for that. I don't have any sympathy for billing for things that weren't done.

But minor scams are, I think, commonplace. Let's take an obstetrical patient who's having a baby. If you came in here and you wanted obstetrical care and you had a normal, uneventful prenatal course, the amount of lab work, or the amount of things like ultrasound, that would be done on you would be relatively minimal, because there's nothing going on.

Now if you have a Medicaid patient who had a similar course, you would be reimbursed about $450 for this prenatal care and delivery. A private fee is about $1,200. So virtually everybody I know, including myself when I was doing Medicaid, would then find some reason or another to do ultrasound, for which you could bill and therefore bring the fee up to around $550 or $600.

An abortion is paid at $140. So by doing three abortions, you would be almost close to receiving what you receive for a normal delivery. Well a delivery, which includes prenatal care, postnatal care, the delivery, and the postop in the hospital, exceeds by a vast amount the energy involved in doing three abortions. So either the therapeutic abortion fee is too high or the delivery fee is too low.

This again opens the door to further abuse that I see going on in the abortion clinics, because in the abortion, if it's done in volume, you can do ten or twelve in an hour, so therefore there is a tremendous economic incentive to line up a large number of these patients. There's no incentive at all to do prenatal care. A patient who needed an abortion could phone up the vast majority of the obstetricians in this area and immediately get it done. The same patient needing prenatal care is limited to probably less than 5 percent, or maybe 10 percent, of practitioners who will accept her.

The practitioner who has a chance from a referral agency to have fifty abortions referred to him a week will be under tremendous pressure to give some kind of a kickback to get these patients, which are what you call gravy or icing on the cake. So there are some built-in factors in the system which lead to abuse.

Condemning the Condemners

Sykes and Matza describe condemning the condemners as a fourth neutralization technique: "The delinquent shifts the focus of attention from his own deviant acts to the motives and behavior of those who disapprove of his violations."[8] This shift enables violators to minimize responsibility for their behavior by construing it as trivial compared to the misdeeds of the rule makers or as rational compared to the irrational expectations of the rule makers.

In a typical condemnation of the Medicaid program, one of our respondents insisted that Medicaid not only invited but demanded cheating:

It's not related to reality, you know. It's done by people who are not medical people, who know nothing about the services being provided. One of the peculiarities that they do is that they make arbitrary decisions about things totally unrelated to the services you provide. They're constantly irritating and aggravating the doctors and their staff.

They say, "What we used to do, we're not going to do anymore." And you're already three months into your new billing system. I could keep you here the rest of the day giving you examples of their kind of idiocy, that they somehow manage to make sense out of in their little peculiar world that's unrelated to ours. They've built in systems that either ask for somebody to cheat, you know, or to cheat the patient on the type of care that's provided. You put somebody in the position where lying is the most reasonable course, and they will lie. The patients will lie; the doctor may even lie on what they say about what happened.

This physician illustrated his point by citing the often-criticized Medicaid rule that three months must elapse between compensable abortions. Suppose, he argued, a young woman had undergone an abortion in his office one week short of three months ago. According to the rules, he should tell her to come back the following week. But suppose she insists that she has to visit her sick mother in another state. This puts "everybody in a position because somebody has made some rule that doesn't make sense." A "naive" doctor would do the young woman "a favor" and postdate the reimbursement form. But, he concluded, "I don't know whether there's any naive doctors around anymore; they've been so hassled and harassed by this system."

That the Medicaid regulations might represent an attempt, however flawed, to control abuse, rather than an effort to harass or second-guess doctors, did not enter into the thinking of doctors who condemned the system as arbitrary, capricious, and unreasonable. One doctor could only fall back on the word "ridiculous":

I think they are ridiculous. We ask permission; we send them proof; we send them everything. One of them even asked me for a picture of the patient. I told him: "Who do you think I am, a crook or what? I am telling you this big long hernia there is hanging out of the testicles." I said: "Well, what do I send a picture of? Oh man, you are crazy." And that's what I do; I sent a picture, but it was absolutely ridiculous.

They are spending so much money. So many secretaries they have. They check all the cases in the hospitals, the Medicaid cases that go in, all the welfare cases they check.

A psychiatrist expressed a similar sense of frustration with what he regarded as petty interference with his professional autonomy: "There is a problem with the number of sessions. You had to make it sound like the person was really in bad shape. And then, they always sent it back, saying, 'Please give us more information,' which is more harassment. So you write it again, and send it in, and often that would be OK'd the second time."

Although the sanctioned physicians focused their scorn on particular aspects of the program that related to their own misconduct, they had fewer complaints about reimbursement levels and "unnecessary" regulation than our comparison group of nonsanctioned physicians. Slightly more than half (57 percent) of the sanctioned physicians felt reimbursement was too low, an opinion shared by 73 percent of the nonsanctioned doctors. And almost two-thirds of the sanctioned physicians (62 percent), compared to only 23 percent of the nonsanctioned, said they had no complaints about unnecessary Medicaid regulations. This pattern of self-serving selective disapproval resembles a phenomenon observed in prison culture, where "common criminals" are notably hostile to child molesters and traitors.[9]

Appeal to Higher Loyalties

The fifth and final neutralization technique discussed by Sykes and Matza is the appeal to higher loyalties. Delinquents engage in lawbreaking, they say, to benefit smaller and more intimate groups to which they belong, such as their gangs or their friendship networks. Laws are broken "because other norms, held to be more pressing or involving a higher loyalty, are accorded precedence."[10] For the sanctioned physicians, such higher loyalties included service to patients and adherence to professional standards. In an unusual case, one physician insisted that being diagnosed with cancer prompted his cheating. He was worried about whether his infant son would have an adequate inheritance. In addition, he said he was despondent, angry, and bitter and wanted to get caught because of a wish to destroy himself or "to get back at the world" for his illness.

A Subculture of Delinquency?

Every sanctioned doctor we interviewed relied on one or more neutralization techniques to explain what had happened, and only rarely did we hear even the most elemental acknowledgment of self-serving motives. The structure of Medicaid, as we have noted, offers more than ample opportunities to harvest rationalizations that locate blame on factors other than the offender's lack of restraint. At times, doctors agreed that they might have been more careful and diligent about supervising others or challenging unusual goings-on, but such admissions were most often accompanied by claims to have been concerned with more important, socially valuable matters. On occasion, we heard physicians suggest that their own stupidity led to their apprehension— but it was the method of cheating, not the cheating itself, that they regretted.

The tenor of the interviews indicated that the cavalier attitudes these doctors had adopted toward the government benefit programs had been at least partially absorbed from others in the profession, and that professional values may effectively neutralize conflicts of conscience. Here we took our cue from Matza's discussion of a "subculture of juvenile delinquency"—"a setting in which the commission of delinquency is common knowledge among a group" and which provides norms and beliefs that "function as the extenuating conditions under which delinquency is permissible."[11] A subculture of medical delinquency, we concluded, arises, thrives, and grows in large part because of the tension between bureaucratic regulation and professional norms of autonomy.

Physicians who cheated government programs were not committed to a life of crime and undoubtedly did not cheat on all their billings. Nor did they always steal from Medicaid or from private insurance programs; they probably were honest in much of their work. But when these doctors did defy Medicaid's legal requirements, they typically offered professional justifications in lieu of defining their activities as deviant, illegal, or criminal.

HOW THEY WERE TREATED

As we have seen, the explanations doctors offered for their criminal activities tended to be mundane—low drama, at best. None described their crimes as a brave political stand against a loathsome bureaucracy or as a blow struck in defense of a glorious cause. Those who portrayed their actions as altruistic did not picture themselves as behaving much differently from any good physician.

The ho-hum tone of their stories altered, however, when they began

to describe how they were treated by the government authorities. De-
picting themselves as victims in modern tragedies, these physicians
recounted tales filled with drama about the authorities' stupefying
overreaction, their insulting attacks on the physicians' self-image and
integrity. Typical of their bitterness about the unfairness of their plight
was the following comment: "I have had my eyes opened up to the ways
of the world. When the government acts, it doesn't let the Constitution
stand in its way. A man can be plucked out of nowhere and shipped to
Siberia. That's how it was with me."

Detection

The doctors' tales of the detections of their offenses reaffirmed what
enforcement agents reported to us. The investigators believe they catch
only the stupid crooks, "the ones who jump into the boat." Many of
the sanctioned physicians seconded this view. One lamented, "It was
the dumbest thing for a psychiatrist to do, because obviously you're
going to get caught. I mean, it comes in on a computer. There's no way
they could miss." He added sarcastically, "That's the only thing I see
as unfair about Medi-Cal—they've got the whole thing fixed so that
psychiatrists are the only ones that get caught."

Detection sometimes resulted from a patient's complaints about a
doctor. A psychiatrist who pled guilty to attempted rape claimed the
charges of impropriety against him were based on groundless accusations by a patient who was angry because he had stopped prescribing
drugs for her. He railed against the patient: "She is a paranoid schizophrenic, and these people have a known statistical proclivity for at-
tacking physicians with false accusations, OK? So this patient has been
on Valium for quite a while, and I decided she was misusing it, or trying
to, and I stopped it. So in her rage, she runs off somewhere else and
she accuses me of sexually abusing her, having raped her a hundred
times."

Another physician also believed she got into trouble only because her
reasonable action had angered an unreasonable patient:

She brought her child in because she swallowed a penny . . . let's say six hours
before. She brought the child in the afternoon, while she swallowed the penny

in the early morning. The secretary saw the child was playing, so she put the child according to the time she came in. I think she was number twelve, something like that.

And I came in and I, of course, do the number one. And the mother said, "Why isn't my child being seen? This is an emergency." So the secretary said, "She's playing. It doesn't look like an emergency. So why don't you wait your turn?" And she left mad.

Well, my secretary probably forgot and put in the invoice because she usually puts the invoices together at the end of the day and hands me the invoices. I charged the patient for an upper respiratory infection because every kid I see always has a cold. Three months later the mom gets a statement.

Of course I never saw the kid. I don't even know if I saw the kid. I saw forty patients that day. Then she came to see the secretary. I wasn't there. She said, "What's this?" The secretary said, "Why don't you sit down and wait, and talk to her?" She didn't wait. I think she went to Medicaid.

We asked this doctor whether she commonly put down "upper respiratory infection" when she could not remember a particular patient's diagnosis; she replied, "Yes, that's safe."

Doctors whose illegal acts were uncovered by sting operations were especially incensed at the government's conduct. Most believed they had been entrapped—lured into the wrongful behaviors by agents provocateurs. Almost all these doctors had come to the attention of law enforcement officers because they had written prescriptions for relatively large quantities of Schedule 2 and Schedule 3 drugs (such as Valium and codeine). But these physicians were highly irritated that the government was allowed to contaminate the doctor-patient relationship. Undercover work, they felt, was an assault on their own trusting natures and forever after made them suspicious about the truth of what patients told them.

The Process

Many of the doctors said it never had occurred to them that their behaviors might arouse the suspicions of government enforcement agents. They told us repeatedly that they knew of no colleagues who had been punished for Medicaid violations. If true, such views may have played into the situation in which these doctors ultimately found themselves. Had they been more aware of enforcement efforts, they might have either obeyed the rules or engaged in the kinds of violations, such as overutilization, that were unlikely to arouse any enforcement reaction.

Almost two-thirds of the sanctioned physicians we interviewed said they understood the Medicaid regulations, but the same proportion reported they were not familiar with the sanctions attached to violations. Many apparently expected that a slap on the wrist would be the worst that would happen to them if apprehended. One physician, for instance, who had been caught for "unknowingly" billing for three visits a month for patients he had been seeing only twice in that period, said he had presumed he would be notified of the discrepancy and allowed to repay the money. In anticipation of benign treatment, most of the doctors freely turned over their files to investigative agents. They were startled when they were presented with indictments rather than invoices.

Several sanctioned doctors had little understanding of criminal law. One, for example, was surprised that the misdemeanor charges against him were handled in criminal court. (Misdemeanors are, by definition, criminal offenses, though less serious than felonies.) Others had expected their reputations as law-abiding citizens to work in their favor. "I even stop for yellow lights," one of them said.

A number of the doctors complained that they, and especially their attorneys, had failed to appreciate the awful consequences that could result from pleading guilty to the charges:

They [the investigators] said, "Well, if you just plead guilty to prescribing medications to a drug user, we will forget the whole thing and drop it." So I said, "All right, I would." I thought it was a very innocuous sort of thing, nolo contendere or that. Well, it turns out that it was not innocuous, because any nolo contendere against a doctor in California can be subject for revocation of his license or disciplinary action by BMQA [the state licensing agency].

When the doctors discovered that pleading guilty would not necessarily result in more lenient treatment, some elected to fight strenuously. As one said about what had happened to colleagues charged with him for similar activities, "The ones who pleaded guilty got more punishment than they thought. That was one of the reasons that I had to fight, because not only did they spend some jail time—in fact, all the ones who pleaded guilty were the ones given jail sentences—they were allowed to serve them on weekends. I think the punishment was extreme."

Not one of the sanctioned physicians had much good to say about his or her attorney. Even the most positive assessment of an attorney was peppered with discontent:

I had two lawyers. The first lawyer did the first part of it. My family, when it came to the second part, said don't get him any more, because they didn't like the results of the first one. So I got this other lawyer, excellent man. I don't think he understood the whole thing, the medical picture. Medicine has a lot of things unique to it. The lawyer has to know about those things in order to be really good and do a great job. He didn't understand a lot of little items, which I think would have improved matters had he.

Another physician's criticisms of his counsel—as well as the entire criminal justice system—sounded much like the gripe of any street criminal: "That's one thing about the whole legal system: There is no justice. You get an attorney; they make deals. Some make deals with you. The D.A. says, 'We want that guy. You get in with us, we will owe you.' They can do it. I had an attorney then. But now, I got sick of attorneys, and don't take anything they say. I was completely displeased; he didn't know anything more than I already knew."

Some doctors decided not to fight the charges against them because of the expense. (Those who put a dollar amount on the cost of their defense quoted $1,000 a day for an attorney.) For physicians who faced a penalty no more severe than suspension from participation in Medicaid, the costs of doing battle did not seem worthwhile; some had voluntarily discontinued accepting Medicaid patients as soon as their problems with the authorities surfaced. Nonetheless, they criticized the government for bypassing due process. One doctor claimed he had not received notice of the nature of his violation and learned of his suspension from a newspaper story. His lawyers then calculated that the cost of fighting the case would far exceed the loss of income associated with suspension from Medicaid. Besides, the doctor maintains, he learned of his suspension so belatedly that it probably would have taken longer to get reinstated than to wait out the remainder of the suspension.

Most of the elderly physicians were particularly cooperative with the investigators and did not fight the charges. Near or past retirement age, they figured they might just as well limit or suspend their practice of medicine.

Punishment

As discussed earlier, some physicians' cases were resolved through administrative procedures, while others were handled in the criminal courts. In both arenas, the punishments varied widely.

Some physicians who served jail terms tended to downplay the seriousness of the consequences and even found some pleasure in the experience, probably because the incarcerations were confined to weekends:

I had to spend weekends out at the minimum security place. This of itself was not such a terrible thing. This can happen to any man picked up for drunk driving. It was called fifteen days and actually it was only ten. You could go in on a Friday around 6 P.M., and they put you in some prison clothes, and get out Sunday evening. So actually you are only there for two nights and two days, but they count it as three days. It was five weekends.

This was very hard on my wife. I took it rather easily, sort of enjoyed it. It was an experience that nobody else could experience unless they got their ass in a bind. Mostly drunks. It was interesting. They had a good library.

In contrast, the most dire punishment was loss of one's medical license. One physician noted that the licensing board had "the real power to kill you." Judges could only put him on probation, confine him, or fine him, but the state medical board could cut off his "lifeblood."

For many doctors, the personal and professional repercussions of the accusations outweighed the official penalties. Many cited the toll of legal costs: "We were going to appeal to the Superior Court. And then I find that for me to appeal, I had to come up with another $7,500 cash just to get the transcript. That says nothing about the cost of the attorney and so forth. By the time we had gone through this, all of it had just drained me down. I almost went bankrupt. I'm just now recovering from it."

Almost three-quarters of the doctors reported that their practices had suffered as a result of their troubles with the government, although 7 percent said their practices had grown, presumably for unrelated reasons. Loss of Medicaid billings was probably the prime factor in declining income, though some doctors pointed to the effects of negative publicity: "They published my name everywhere. It's enormously embarrassing because I've got a pretty good reputation. I depended entirely on other doctors' referrals. They see me listed amongst all those yo-yos."

A handful of doctors alluded to the deterioration of their marriages and the difficulties experienced by their children as consequences of the publicity given to their cases. One doctor's wife had left the country with the children, who, he said, "were coming home from school in tears," having been told by playmates, "'Your dad is a crook and should be in prison.'" Another physician said he had been forced to relocate to a much less desirable town after the Medicaid case against him: "We had to move from an area we all loved to an area where economically it's great, but how would you like to live here? I feel like I'm in exile. I have very little in common with the people here. The ones that were hurt the most were my children. One in particular would have turned out much better had we stayed. All his old friends are achieving something, and he's not."

Another doctor reported having become disenchanted with medicine and passingly entertaining the idea of becoming a lawyer:

My goals have changed. My joke to my patients has always been: "I want to die on the way to work or on the way home from work." But now, I'm sliding to the fact of maybe retiring. I've even thought of going into law, and I dislike lawyers. But medicine does not have the kind of things that I fell in love with at first. I get the feeling it has become more business than medicine. That annoys me. The fact that they are not paying me enough to really be comfortable; so that I have been considering some teaching positions.

Others merely maintained that they had been disabused of their earlier "do-gooder" attitude toward Medicaid patients and now despised them. But one physician had a much more wrenching verdict on his experience: "It's the end of the world for the doctor who's been knocked down by the government. It's the end of the world. He might as well die."

ATTITUDES TOWARD MEDICAID, FRAUD, AND ABUSE

We had hoped that respondents might be able to shed some light on the actual extent of Medicaid fraud and abuse. But one-third of the doctors had no idea how much cheating was going on, another third felt there was very little cheating, 10 percent felt there was a moderate amount, and about 25 percent believed there were a lot of violations. The consensus was split between two positions: One group believed that a great many doctors were cheating the government and that they had been picked out of the crowd, while the other group believed that Medicaid crime was a relatively small problem being overblown by the authorities and that their own misdeeds were relatively insignificant. Estimates of the prevalence of fraud given by the sanctioned doctors and the nonsanctioned comparison group differed at a level of statistical significance; sanctioned doctors reported higher figures.

Asked about conditions that contribute to Medicaid fraud, doctors often focused on matters directly related to their own cases. Doctors in the sanctioned group often noted the ease with which offenses could be committed as a major factor in their difficulties—a recurrent theme in all commentaries about the Medicaid program. One doctor put it quite succinctly: "We are all human beings, and given the right temptations, we will all succumb." Another doctor, who had been proceeded against, wished he had been warned of the temptations: "Most of us fellows would have really profited by just somebody from the system to tell us, 'We know these temptations are around, but don't you guys get trapped into it.' But nobody bothered to even tell us these laws had been passed."

But ignorance of the law was not the sanctioned physicians' main problem: 61 percent of the sanctioned physicians reported they were fully aware of the regulations at the time of their violations; only 46 percent of the nonsanctioned doctors reported similar knowledge. According to the sanctioned doctors, deterrence tactics should focus on increasing physicians' awareness of the penalties for Medicaid violations. One doctor advised, "One way [to deter others] would be when a new physician enrolls in the program, to send some case vignettes— ways in which transgressions have occurred and the penalties that resulted." A lack of awareness about the penalties among the physicians in our sample comparison group was pronounced. Almost two-thirds of the sanctioned group, compared to only 9 percent of the nonsanctioned physicians, felt that punishment was likely for some providers, although few members of either group felt that sanctions for Medicaid wrongdoing were very likely.

"Deterrence research," writes Johannes Andenaes, "has been mainly concerned with the effects of severity and certainty of sanctions." He suggests a third factor as well: "the perceived legitimacy of the criminal justice system and of the particular statute under examination." Andenaes argues that "to exert a moral influence, the law and the machinery for enforcement of it must be looked upon as wielding legitimate authority," and concludes that "a more lenient system, which is accepted as fair and consistent, has a stronger impact than a more severe system which creates the impression of inconsistency and arbitrariness."[12]

The physicians' widespread dissatisfaction with Medicaid covered much ground, but the crucial issue was the intrusion of a third party into the relationship between physician and patient. (This criticism obviously applies to private insurance, but we did not explore this matter.) A representative comment: "Third-party medicine is unacceptable to me because the third party always speaks from the standpoint of its own vested interest. It never really speaks for the interest of the physicians, and hardly speaks for the interest of the patient." Another physician repeated this point:

In general, because of the intervention of the third party, cost of minimal care has become so high that nobody can afford it, unless you are Getty. You have to have third-party insurance, but it has changed medical care to a large extent. Let's say I go in at 2 o'clock in the morning and some guy is bleeding to death of an ulcer. I save his life. I see him once or twice in the office. Six months later he doesn't even know my name. He never got a bill. The insurance company got the bill, the insurance company paid me. He doesn't even know me. And that's disappointing.

Also surprisingly for us, there was no significant difference between members of the two groups about whether the programs were "legit-imate." We had expected the sanctioned doctors to hide more often behind a program-blaming stance. More than half of each group, however, did not regard the programs as legitimate medical operations; only 10 percent took the opposite viewpoint.

Both sanctioned and nonsanctioned doctors overwhelmingly indi-cated the Medicaid program was not fair, and the nonsanctioned group was even more negative than the sanctioned doctors. As one nonsanc-tioned physician said, "It's like tying someone's hands and telling them to lift a big rock." The sanctioned doctors tended to support the need for regulations but indicated that more of the control should come from the medical profession itself rather than from the government.

Finally, we observed a statistically significant difference ($p < .05$) in the responses of sanctioned and nonsanctioned physicians regarding their views of the consistency of enforcement efforts. Sanctioned phy-sicians, as might be expected, saw enforcement as inconsistent (74 percent); those who had not been sanctioned were almost evenly split among the response categories: consistent (30 percent), inconsistent (38 percent), don't know (32 percent). Both groups cited similar types of inconsistencies: bias against certain specialties (33 percent), bias against big vendors (28 percent), and bias against minorities (23 percent). Other sources of inconsistency included biases against urban doctors and solo practitioners, taking the easiest cases, and politics; together, these ac-counted for an additional 18 percent of the responses.

CONCLUSION

The establishment of the Medicaid program provided new opportunities for doctors and other medical practitioners and organizations to commit criminal acts and to violate administrative regulations. Our research did not yield a composite portrait of physicians who typically get into trouble with Medicaid, though there are some recurring traits in the roster of physicians dealt with by the authorities. The stereotypical image of the violator as an inner-city doctor associated with a Medicaid mill is misleading: Offenders include some of the most respectable members of the profession and physicians of all ages, specialties, and attitudes toward patients and government medical benefit programs.

Chapter Six

Conclusions and Speculations

The case histories of frauds perpetrated by physicians against Medicaid illustrate that doctors, however highly regarded or well off, are no exception to the general principle that in a culture in which material wealth is highly valued, some persons who appear to have no reasonable need to do so will break the law in order to obtain extra money. The renowned nineteenth-century sociologist Emile Durkheim looked to the particular form of discontent among affluent, powerful persons to explain their feeling that ordinary limits did not apply to them: "Wealth, by the power it bestows, deceives us into believing that we depend on ourselves only. Reducing the resistance we encounter from objects, it suggests the possibility of unlimited success against them. The less limited one feels, the more intolerable all limitations appear."[1]

The widespread malaise created in the ranks of the medical profession by the intrusion of the government into how doctors practice and charge for their services has spawned among some practitioners a truculent disregard of the rules under which Medicaid work is to be done. The conditions that facilitate this kind of fraud include (1) the perpetrator's ability to redefine the violation, both in private and to others, in benign terms; (2) the perpetrator's feeling that insensitive external forces are interfering with his or her just deserts; (3) the availability of opportunities to violate the law easily; and (4) the perpetrator's belief that the violations are unlikely to be discovered or, if found out, are unlikely to result in serious penalties.

Government regulation of medical benefit programs not only cuts deeply into physicians' autonomy but also limits their ability to maximize their incomes. Few, if any, physicians enter medicine intending to make a fortune by violating the regulations, but the promise of a healthy income is an incentive for embarking on a long, arduous period of training. And the government medical benefit programs provide an enticing array of opportunities for financial self-aggrandizement. Above all, they have dramatically reduced one of the most powerful deterrents to crime, especially for middle- and upper-class perpetrators: the sense of guilt and the force of conscience associated with depredations against known human victims. The programs also defused a second forceful deterrent: they made it easy to commit violations. All a doctor (or a billing clerk) needs to do is check off a more expensive procedure than the one that was performed; in the course of a year, such "upgrades" can generate thousands of extra dollars.

Physicians are expected to place patients' welfare above their own interests and are specifically prohibited from engaging in business practices that are acceptable in other professions.[2] But the pressure to practice medicine in a manner that yields the highest financial return can be quite strong, especially if patients' health is not compromised by billing scams. Nor are all doctors immune from the temptation to compromise care for financial gain. In an editorial, for example, in the *New England Journal of Medicine* Arnold Relman argued for legislation banning physicians from selling prescription drugs to their patients for profit, which he cited as a conflict of interest. To maintain or increase their incomes, Relman writes, physicians "may succumb to the temptation to overprescribe or prescribe a drug they have in their necessarily limited stock, whether or not it is the most appropriate treatment for the patient." Implicit in Relman's appeal for legislation is the caution that professional ethics alone do not protect patients:

Physicians are not primarily vendors, but counselors and fiduciaries on whom patients rely for advice. When doctors profit by selling their patients drugs that they themselves have prescribed, they are attempting to fill two basically incompatible roles—those of fiduciary and vendor. This bill is necessary to protect the public from possible abuse resulting from the confusion of these roles and to make clear that we want our doctors to act as protectors of their patients' interests and not as ordinary tradespeople.[3]

Unnecessary X rays are another example of unethical conduct motivated by a financial calculus. A doctor recently told us that he now placed much greater emphasis on X raying as many patients as possible because insurance payments on X rays were particularly good in terms of the investment of staff time and the expense of the equipment. This is the kind of cost-benefit analysis any fiscally sensible entrepreneur might make, but the public expects doctors to stand apart from and above the business crowd and to dedicate their sophisticated skills and insights to the public welfare. As we noted in chapter 1, Talcott Parsons correctly ascertained that for the medical profession to remain autonomous, its members have to practice selflessly, or at least be perceived to do so. In the long run, Parsons argued, altruism would serve physicians' best interests.[4] Through the power of their professional organizations, doctors were able to attain a monopoly on services deemed essential by a client population that often could rely for payments on the very deep pockets of insurers. The temptation to dip their hands as far as possible into those pockets, however, proved irresistible to some physicians. The outcome seems to be fashioning a contemporary updating of the cautionary tale of killing the goose that lays the golden eggs.

Medicaid has played a major role in altering the public's image of the physician as a selfless professional. By delivering free or inexpensive service to the poor, doctors—primarily white, male doctors—maintained the altruistic image necessary to ensure physician autonomy. Medicaid expanded the medical market by paying for care for the poor. The program eventually created a new class of doctors—many of them from minority groups and with training at foreign medical schools—who filled the gap when more successful practitioners either turned their backs on Medicaid or, as they made their way upward, withdrew from it. By simultaneously expanding the number of hospitals and keeping medical school enrollments down, American medical policy has produced, according to one analyst, "a new lower tier in the medical profession drawn from the Third World," thereby making medicine one of the most ethnically diverse of the upper-income professions in the

United States. But some members of the public appear to be skeptical about the abilities of the one-fifth of American doctors who were born and trained abroad.[5]

The pace of technological change has also affected the public's view of the medical profession. Writing in the early 1950s, Parsons, for example, noted the result of changing medical fashion, which brings first one treatment, and then another, into medical favor: "A technical innovation in the medical field will for a time be slow in 'catching on.' When, however, it begins to be accepted, it will spread very rapidly and be utilized on almost every possible occasion where [any] plausible case for it can be made. This continues until the point is reached where it becomes 'oversold' and a reaction sets in."[6]

In earlier times, when technology developed more slowly, the medical elite was more conservative in adopting new treatments, so as not to threaten the social and economic gains doctors had made. Today new treatments come at us with dizzying regularity and dazzling corporate fanfare by the pharmaceutical industry and others, and the medical profession is suspected of selfishness when new techniques prove of questionable value (such as treatments for baldness) or cause injury or death (as Oraflex did).

We have traced the reasons why, particularly in the early days of Medicaid, the government was hesitant to tighten up the structural constraints that might have reduced the cost of the program. The basic explanation lies in political expediency. To achieve the program's idealistic goal—the best health care for the most people—the architects of Medicaid catered to the demands of the medical lobby. As Joseph Ripple, a political scientist, notes, federal intervention per se did not produce problems; intervention may have been a necessary cause, but it was not a sufficient one. Rather, Ripple points out, the crux of Medicaid's failure is that "the money is thrown into a chaotic, greed-driven system by formulas designed to make it politically acceptable to physicians."[7] As a result, Medicaid inevitably deteriorated to the point where structural reforms became necessary, but these reforms themselves only generated new forms of resistance from within the medical community. Nonetheless, the inexorable direction of reform has been toward a diminution of physicians' power.

Public hostility to physicians and the nation's system of health care delivery has provided the government with a strong base of political support for its incursions against doctors' autonomy. Part of that hostility, of course, has been created by the government itself, as it sought to control health care costs. A survey conducted by the AMA in 1984 documented the public's dissatisfaction and mistrust: 54 percent of the respondents said physicians do not care about people as much as they used to; 67 percent thought doctors were too busy making money; 68 percent said people are losing faith in medicine; only 27 percent thought physicians' fees were reasonable.[8] Alain Enthoven, a professor of management at the Stanford University School of Business, summarizes the litany of complaints with the blunt conclusion that "our health care system is becoming a disaster," even though expenditures for health care equal the total allocated for national defense and education. Uwe Reinhardt, an economist at Princeton University, has declared that the United States now has "a health policy that might be judged comical if it were not so tragic."[9]

Doctors today face the searing scorn and ridicule of gadflies and satirists, a sure sign of vulnerability. How do you decide where to send a patient, columnist Art Buchwald asks Dr. Wesley Heights, part owner of the Kidney Stone Memorial Hospital. "It's strictly a medical decision," the physician replies. "If they have a good health insurance plan, I put them in Kidney Stone. If they don't, I find a bed at Sisters of Mercy. . . . I've been able to look at medical care not only from the patient's viewpoint, but also from the stockholders'. . . . This has made me a better doctor, and richer for the experience."[10]

Certainly the United States will not abandon the commitment to health care for the poor. Should Medicaid become hopelessly unable to deliver quality care at a reasonable price, new programs will be established to provide care for the destitute, the working poor who do not qualify for Medicaid, and others who have no private medical insurance. In periods of transition, such as now exist, before a new approach and boundaries of behavior are specifically defined, deviance is likely to flourish; and it has been marked in the first decades of Medicaid.

IMPAIRMENT AS A CAUSE OF
WHITE-COLLAR CRIMES

There are those who will commit a crime when to do so requires a good deal of resolve and daring. And there are others—such as most of those who commit Medicaid fraud and abuse—who will violate the law only when it is easy and safe to do so. In other words, no matter how well monitored a program may be and how risky the crime, some physicians will undertake it; at the same time, no matter how easy such fraud might prove to be, some physicians will not cheat. Finally, others will do so only for what they can define as altruistic or otherwise laudable motives. Along this continuum, cheating undoubtedly will vary in a direct relationship to the ease with which it can be done and the presumed pressures on the participants to do so.

In trying to explain why some physicians cheat and others do not, one cannot easily separate personal traits from situational variables. This fact limits our ability to suggest solutions for physician fraud and abuse in Medicaid. The medical model of criminality holds that individual deviation is the cause of lawbreaking activities and that the treatment of offenders must therefore be individualized. Under this rubric, criminal physicians are viewed as "impaired." The "impaired physician" thus represents the profession's medicalization of its members' deviance: The criminal activity is a symptom of psychological disease, and it should be addressed by therapeutic, not penal, means.

One well-known measure of impairment is the widespread use and abuse of drugs by physicians. Conservative estimates place their addiction rate at 1 percent; others suggest that as many as 10 percent of doctors will be less effective because of drug use sometime during their careers. The addiction rate among doctors outdistances that for all other professions—a finding believed to result from a ready availability of drugs that leads to self-treatment for a variety of problems, including pain, fatigue, insomnia, and stress. [11]

Treatment for substance-abusing physicians usually consists of psychotherapy, since—as researchers Hubert Wallot and Jean Lambert point out—"drug addiction [is believed to be] a homogeneous psycho-pathology, mainly a personality disorder presenting passive and psy-chopathic traits as well as oral character." More recent work has rec-ognized that drug addiction among doctors may have a variety of nonpsychological causes and can be described as a public health prob-lem. But research continues to focus on the individual, rather than on social or political factors. Wallot and Lambert, for example, note that "the apparent diversity among physician addicts suggests that we should consider different treatments for a variety of addictive conditions" and that "a typology of the physician addict" is needed. [12]

According to the medical model, individual pathology also plays a role in motivating Medicaid offenses by physicians. We cannot exclude the possibility, for example, that the overrepresentation of psychiatrists in our criminal sample is due to individual differences between psy-chiatrists and other medical practitioners. Several studies suggest such differences do exist: Medical students have reported that psychiatrists appear more emotionally unstable than their other teachers; University of Colorado medical students characterized psychiatrists as compli-cated, temperamental, and emotional; among a sample of British med-ical students, half held negative attitudes about the emotional stability of psychiatrists. [13]

Psychiatric training itself may also contribute to professional devi-ance. According to Donald Light, an academic in the field, psychiatric residents have a high rate of psychopathology, and "the profession is worried about the prevalence." But he speculates that such pathologies may be caused in part by medical education in which psychiatric students learn to "empathize with the patients' craziness." Light argues that "an intense professional training which aims to elicit and give expression to such feelings may well produce emotional disturbances and sanction neurotic mannerisms." [14]

Such observations in no way absolve psychiatrists from personal responsibility for their misconduct; the issue is rather whether psychi-atry's professional structure and norms help shape the forms deviance takes. Are certain types of abuses more likely to occur because psychi-atrists are trained to prescribe psychotropic drugs to alleviate mood disorders? because they have the power to withhold or supply drugs, and to define patients as needing institutional care? because they form uncommonly close relationships with patients?[15]

If individual deviation is, as the medical model holds, the major cause of physicians' crimes, we can expect little change, as the psychological problems of medical students are unlikely to be addressed soon. A study conducted in the early 1980s of medical schools' approaches to preventing physician impairment revealed that most schools had undertaken only minimal efforts.[16]

WOMEN DOCTORS

One major change that might affect the profile of physicians' conduct is the increase in women students at medical schools. At the turn of the twentieth century, women accounted for about 6 percent of America's physicians. In 1910 the Flexner report led to the closing of inferior medical schools, and many of these were women's colleges; so by 1940 the proportion of women in medicine had dropped to 4.4 percent. It rose during World War II and reached 6 percent again by the war's end. Today about 20 percent of all doctors in the United States are women, and women constituted 38 percent of the 1988–89 entering class in the country's 127 medical schools.[17]

Women are greatly underrepresented on the nation's roster of criminal offenders. Common explanations focus on women's socialization and learned fear of the shameful consequences of nontraditional behavior. The advent of the feminist movement has spurred speculation about whether equal opportunity in the workplace would translate into equal opportunities for white-collar crime. The reflex assumption was that as women moved more freely into politics, the professions, and business, they would begin to duplicate the white-collar criminal activities of their male colleagues.[18] The best-known statement of this theme comes from Rita Simon: "As women increase their participation in the labor force, their opportunity to commit certain types of crimes also increases. This explanation assumes that women have no greater store of morality than do men. Their propensities to commit crimes do not differ, but, in the past, their opportunities have been much more limited. As women's opportunities to commit crimes increase . . . , the types of crimes they commit will much more closely resemble those committed by men."[19]

Whether women do or do not have a stronger moral ethic than men is, of course, arguable, as is the idea that women will exploit the opportunities afforded by the workplace. In all quarters, women continue to manifest considerably lower rates of violent criminal acts than men, although when inhibitions are lowered by chronic psychosis, sex role differences in rates of violent behavior in mental hospitals disappear.[20]

The argument has also been made that when women move into more prominent social roles, they bring with them a nurturing, collaborative, cooperative spirit that mediates the aggressiveness and self-interest that motivate male criminals. Best known is Carol Gilligan's thesis that men and women have distinctively different moral orientations. Gilligan asserts that women conceptualize moral questions as problems of care involving empathy and compassion, while men see such problems as matters of rights. Studies in the workplace have found women to be more concerned with helping people, and men more interested in advancement; men also enjoy workplace ruses, hoaxes, and other deceptions more than women do. More particularly, a survey of medical students in North Carolina found that graduating women were less conservative than males and more oriented to humanitarian patient care values and political-economic change in medicine. The author concluded that "women are not yet joining the melting pot of medical conservatism."[21] (Even in sixteenth-century Venice, male and female healers had different approaches: "Though there were obvious exceptions, men were basically concerned simply with gain, acquiring for themselves either money, women, or both. The motives [for women] were more varied and complex.")[22]

Medical historian Paul Starr believes that women have effected changes in the consciousness of the medical profession that may have a bearing on the general ethos of practice:

The older generation of women physicians felt obliged to prove that they could make it on the terms set by the dominant male physicians. The younger generation of women physicians demanded that male physicians change their attitudes and behavior and modify institutional practices to accommodate their needs as women. Here the new consciousness of rights invaded the house of medicine and insisted on changes in the rules of professional behavior and practice.[23]

But Starr offers no evidence for this conclusion, and it seems debatable whether medicine has undergone fundamental structural changes to accommodate women physicians or whether women physicians have tended to enter those occupational niches where their needs might be most satisfactorily met, for example, pediatrics, women's health, addiction disorders, and geriatrics.

Compared to men physicians, women physicians work fewer hours a week, are less likely to belong to the AMA, and are less likely to be sued for malpractice—statistics that may indicate that women physicians take a more relaxed (and perhaps therefore more law-abiding) approach to their work.[24] But the suicide rate among women physicians is higher than that of men physicians and four times higher than the suicide rate for women overall. One research team posed a theory of self-selection—"there is (or has been) some association between affective disorder and the selection of medical education as a career by U.S. women"—and hypothesized that as more women enter medical school, a smaller percentage might be so "laden."[25] But we are much more inclined to see the suicide rate as reflecting women doctors' work experiences rather than their preexisting pathologies. Perhaps they are overwhelmed by the suffering they see, or by the demands of the job combined with family responsibilities, or by sexual harassment at work or blocked professional opportunities.[26]

Women Doctors and Medicaid Fraud

Our count of Medicaid violations does not support the hypothesis that a large influx of women into the medical profession will significantly reduce overall rates of fraud and abuse. Of the 147 violators identified in chapter 4 for whom we could determine gender, 131 were men and 14 were women—proportions that roughly equaled the composition of the profession at the time. That women (and younger) physicians have the highest participation rates in Medicaid may have inflated their presence in our sample.[27] In a sample of 196 physicians convicted for Medi-Cal fraud in California over a seven-year period, 50 of the doctors (or 25 percent) were women. During the same period, about 15 percent of all doctors in the United States, and 12 percent in California, were women.

These results, clearly, are tentative, and much more extensive and sophisticated research remains to be done. Most important, we need time series analyses that take account of the total number of women doctors at work in a given year, their specialties (women are overrepresented in internal medicine and pediatrics and greatly underrepresented in surgery), their level of participation in Medicaid work, their ages, kinds of practice (women physicians are less often self-employed than men doctors), and similar variables.[28]

Several factors would seem to mitigate against Medicaid fraud by women physicians, but these also require further scrutiny. First, because 80 percent of women doctors are married to working professionals, they might not feel pressured to maximize their earnings through cheating. Such pressure is relevant because women—but not men—who commit embezzlement and larceny offenses consistently cite family needs as their motivation. Women doctors also report that, because of less pressure for earnings, they are able to spend more time with individual patients. However, in several surveys women physicians who have children almost invariably report that they have almost total responsibility for child care—a stress not shared by their men colleagues.

Second, the high rates of alcoholism and suicide among women physicians suggest that, more so than their men colleagues, they tend to take their frustrations out on themselves rather than to become physically or fiscally aggressive against others. There also has been some speculation that women who are high achievers are subject to unusual anxiety because of their defiance of traditional role expectations.[29] Both these factors would tend to dampen lawbreaking activities.

If thorough scrutiny of the records of Medicaid violators were to demonstrate few differences between women and men, that might constitute evidence that the lure of Medicaid's fee-for-service structure is sufficiently strong to induce women into lawbreaking. Alternatively, one could argue that women who choose to become doctors have already transcended traditional gender restraints, including those regarding conformity to legal dictates. But if women physicians prove to be significantly less likely to violate Medicaid regulations, then one could not wholly blame the structure of Medicaid—no matter how faulty it may appear—for inciting lawlessness among doctors.

MAKING THE PUNISHMENT
FIT THE CRIME
Delicensing as a Sanction

State medical regulatory boards often resist revoking a physician's license unless the most egregious behavior has been proved. Medicaid violations, when brought to the attention of the licensing authorities at all, are likely to be regarded as peccadilloes, much in the nature of mildly embarrassing pranks. Because Medicaid crimes primarily involve money, they are viewed as irrelevant to the essence of medical practice, which resides in the physical and mental well-being of the patient, not the fiscal integrity of state and federal programs.

An argument can be made for this view. Crooked doctors may be neither better nor worse than their colleagues in their ability to practice medicine effectively. Medical skills are learned only through a long, expensive period of training, and licensing boards apparently assume it would be wasteful to discard a doctor who remains capable of contributing to the community.

Such a benign attitude, however, rarely prevails in other occupations regulated by the state. Teachers, for instance, typically are reported to their school district if they are apprehended for drunkenness or other unseemly or illegal behavior, on the assumption that such conduct bodes poorly for classroom performance and destroys the teachers' usefulness as role models for students. Erring teachers in California are likely to be "requested" to surrender their licenses or face an administrative procedure that, they are artfully led to understand, will prove both expensive and embarrassing. Most teachers take the hint, especially if it is accompanied by the carrot that they might, if they go quietly now, regain their license after a decent interval.[30]

Physicians violating Medicaid statutes only infrequently encounter such pressure from their professional regulatory boards, and only when the precipitating incidents are far more serious than overservicing or cheating on Medicaid billings. But disciplinary actions against physicians have been increasing, probably because of the profession's desire to keep its house somewhat clean in order to obtain tort reforms. But problems and wrongdoing continue apace. In 1985 the AMA conservatively judged that 10,000 physicians were alcoholics and 4,000 drug addicts. In 1987 the medical director of the Committee for Physicians Health estimated that 4,000 of New York's 45,000 doctors "were at some stage of chemical dependence," and hundreds more were emotionally or mentally ill. Estimates supplied to congressional committees suggest that between 5 and 10 percent of U.S. doctors are impaired.[31] Other studies show that some physicians should never have been licensed at all. Investigations by state officials, the National Board of Medical Examiners, and the Federal Bureau of Investigation have uncovered a large number of licensing test violations. Up to $50,000 purportedly was paid for an advance copy of the test, and applicants have used crib sheets and paid others to take the exam in their place. In 1983 somewhere between 3,000 and 4,000 of the 17,000 graduates of overseas medical schools who sat for a qualifying examination for U.S. internships and residencies had seen copies of the test before it was administered at centers in Mexico, Canada, the Caribbean, and the United States. In 1985 a congressional health subcommittee report estimated that 10,000 physicians in the United States did not attend medical school but paid from $5,000 to $25,000 for fake diplomas.[32]

An investigation by California's medical licensing board discovered that few of the 2,600 graduates of overseas medical schools applying for medical licenses in that state had offered sufficient documentation, and that the documentation submitted was "often misleading or fraudulent." Across the country, state licensing officials believe that more than 28,000 unlicensed and untrained persons may be practicing medicine.[33]

Each state's oversight board is somewhat differently constituted, but most possess broad authority to license and discipline physicians within their borders. The vast majority of board members are physicians, usually appointed by the governor or the state medical society. In a typical year, the state boards across the country take action against more than 2,000 doctors—about twice as many as in the early 1980s—not including impaired physicians undergoing treatment as part of a voluntary agreement with the board. States vary dramatically in their imposition of revocations, suspensions, and probations. In 1989 West Virginia disciplined 8.6 physicians per 1,000, Kansas, only 0.45 per 1,000. Dr. Sidney Wolfe, director of the Health Research Group, a Nader affiliate, maintained, "A physician can still operate drunk, commit a gross act of negligence or sexually assault a patient and receive a mere slap on the wrist." Wolfe estimates that more than 100,000 Americans are injured or killed each year as a result of doctors' negligence.[34]

There are specific weaknesses throughout the sanctioning process. A doctor whose work is deemed unsatisfactory by a hospital peer review group may be allowed to resign from the staff. Unlike dismissals for cause, these resignations need not be reported to the state licensing board.[35] Until the recent inauguration of a nationwide computer database of disciplinary actions against physicians, many who had been barred by state boards were able to continue their practice by moving to another state because states often failed to report problem doctors to the Federation of State Medical Boards (FSMB), a private clearinghouse for such information. Nor in the past did the AMA take any steps to inform states of adverse actions against physicians' licenses, arguing it feared lawsuits.

In 1984, for example, a study by the General Accounting Office found that 33 of 181 medical doctors and doctors of osteopathy whose licenses had been revoked in Ohio, Pennsylvania, and Michigan between 1977 and 1982 had moved to another state and resumed their practices. Because many of the defrocked doctors already held licenses in the states to which they relocated, they could open shop immediately upon arrival, without any potentially embarrassing paperwork. An osteopath, for example, had been convicted of mail fraud and false representation in Pennsylvania for filing false claims. He served a prison term, agreed to repay the federal government $150,000, and lost his licenses in Pennsylvania and Virginia. But when he was released, he set up a practice in Vanceburg, Kentucky, and three years passed before Kentucky authorities learned of his conviction. A few months after the Kentucky board voted to place him on probation for five years, he left the state.[36]

Problem physicians have also been able to escape into the military, which does not require its doctors to hold medical licenses. About 21 percent of the approximately 13,000 service physicians are not licensed. While most probably let their licenses lapse after entering the military or joined the service immediately after completing medical school, some had had licensing problems.[37]

It is too soon to evaluate the effectiveness of the National Practitioner Data Bank—popularly known as "doc in a box"—which went on line in September 1990. The bank, estimated to cost $15.9 million, tracks both malpractice actions and disciplinary proceedings against licensed health care practitioners. Providers of information are granted immunity from lawsuits by those whose names they forward. Hospitals are required to report doctors who resign after an investigation of them was started, and hospitals are required to consult the registry at least once every two years regarding present and prospective personnel. The registry is not retroactive and is not available to the public.[38]

The Medical Profession's Response

The *New England Journal of Medicine* has noted that the absence of forceful state disciplinary action has lent "credence to popular suspicions that the medical boards have not been dealing effectively with this problem."[39] Daniel Ein, a physician in the District of Columbia, argued that the profession must change its members' attitudes about self-monitoring: "Physicians, long reluctant to criticize each other, have an ethical responsibility to protect the public from unscrupulous and incompetent practitioners. Grievance mechanisms against physicians already exist within medical societies. Their availability must be more widely publicized. Licensing agencies must be given the resources to investigate claims adequately and mete out punishments."[40]

In recent years, the medical profession has been pressed to rid its ranks of problem physicians in exchange for malpractice tort reforms.

An executive vice-president of the AMA, during an interview with us, expressed the association's new line of thinking about professional responsibility: "We want to make sure that the mechanisms are in place to deal with whatever number of deviant, dishonest, or incompetent doctors are out there. We want the physicians to have confidence in the disciplinary mechanisms so that a reasonably competent doctor should not fear a disciplinary mechanism. We want something that will document the competence. We want something that will instill confidence in the physicians who deal with it. And we want something that is publicly identifiable as accountability."

This new enthusiasm about disciplinary procedures may also be related to concerns about a glut, or at least a surplus, of physicians. The number of physicians in the United States has increased from 14 per 10,000 people at the end of World War II, to 17 per 10,000 in 1976, and 22 per 10,000 in 1987. (In some parts of the country, underworked doctors have even resumed making housecalls.)[41] Among the specialties that have become particularly overcrowded is surgery. In 1981 the United States had a surplus of 30,000 to 40,000 surgeons, and their ranks have continued to soar.[42]

The demand for medical services, however, appears to be tightening. Up through the 1980s Medicare and Medicaid fueled an increase in demand. But now corporations have begun to shop around for the best health care deal, and enrollments in health maintenance organizations (HMOs) are also dampening demand. The AMA's response has been an entrepreneurial one. The association has called for medical schools to decrease their enrollments—rather than proposing a plan that would encourage "surplus" doctors to practice in communities that have too few health care providers.

THE TRANSFORMATION OF
AMERICAN MEDICINE

In his excellent history of American medicine, Paul Starr describes how the medical profession over time turned its scientific knowledge and authority into social privilege, economic power, and political influence. But today that authority and power are being eroded by HMOs, which introduce a competitive form of bureaucratic organization into medical care. Insurance companies, also under pressure to control costs, are striving for new methods to regulate medical decisions. At the same time, hospitals and other health care facilities have been merging into larger and more powerful corporate systems. In the background looms the regulatory power of the state and federal governments; in the foreground, the stunning decline in the public's opinion of physicians. "Increasingly, over the past decade," Starr writes, "philosophers, lawyers, sociologists, historians, and feminists . . . have portrayed the medical profession as a dominating, monopolizing, self-interested force. Once a hero, the doctor has now become a villain."[43]

Starr thus foresees an inevitable decline in the professional suzerainty physicians enjoy. As corporate forces continue to move into key management roles in medicine, doctors lose their aura and become employees whose most essential contribution is to the well-being of the organization itself:

The great irony is that the opposition of doctors and hospitals to public control of public programs set in motion entrepreneurial forces that may end up depriving both public doctors and local voluntary hospitals of their traditional autonomy.

A corporate sector in health care is also likely to aggravate inequalities in access to health care. Profit-making enterprises are not interested in treating those who cannot pay. The voluntary hospital may not treat the poor the same as the rich, but they do treat them and often treat them well. A system in which corporate enterprises play a larger part is likely to be more segmented and stratified. With cutbacks in public financing coming at the same time, the two-class system in medical care is likely to become only more conspicuous.[44]

If corporate control comes to dominate American health care, medical fraud and abuse undoubtedly will change. For when doctors are salaried employees, they have no financial incentive to cheat unless the company sets production quotas that must be achieved or matches salaries to production. Under a corporate system, moreover, doctors' decision-making powers may be so curtailed that, like nurses, they are much of the time obligated to do no more than carry out regulations. (Nurses rarely show up as Medicaid violators, and then as accomplices to a physician's schemes.) Nonetheless, as a researcher in the field points out, although "individual physicians may lose control over for-profit hospitals and the more general growth of a capitalistic structure and mentality within medicine, such a loss is not inevitable." Unlike most other employees, physicians remain capable of imposing their own rules on those for whom they presumably work; in Ritzer's words, doctors are "both constrained by the new structural realities in medicine and simultaneously creating, recreating and even changing these structures."[45]

In the face of corporate pressures, some physicians are warming up to the prospect of some form of national health insurance. Indeed, both Uwe Reinhardt, an economist, and Dr. Philip Lee, head of the Institute of Health Policy Studies at the University of California, San Francisco, believe that physicians will become the leading advocates of national health insurance because they will come to see it as the best financial deal they can cut.[46]

The general public has already been persuaded: In a Harris poll conducted in 1989, an overwhelming 91 percent of respondents agreed that "every American should have the right to get the best possible health care—as good as the treatment a millionaire gets." And to achieve this result, 63 percent favored a government-funded national health plan.[47] Today, however, some 37 million Americans (about one-third of them children) lack health coverage of any kind, and the United States remains the only industrialized nation in the world, except South Africa, that does not have a national health insurance program.

Nonetheless, doctors have generally been more sanguine than the public at large in their assessment of the health care system. A Harris survey conducted in 1982 found that 68 percent of physicians who headed organized medical groups and 48 percent of doctors—compared to just 21 percent of the general public—thought the American medical system was operating "pretty well" and needed only "minor changes." Only 3 percent of the physicians agreed with a view held by 25 percent of the general public that there was so much wrong with the American health care system that it needed complete restructuring. Similarly, 61 percent of the public, but only 13 percent of the practicing physicians, believed that government price controls on doctors and hospital fees were desirable. Almost half the physicians, however, believed that basic changes were needed in the medical *insurance* system.[48]

To the debate over national health insurance, we offer one caveat regarding the forms of medical service delivery and their effects on quality of care. An HMO system provides structural temptations to offer inadequate service to patients. The threat of tort suits by private parties may, in part, control the undertreatment; but unless a supervising government agency establishes guidelines on what must be done for which kinds of patients, and enforces strong penalties for undertreatment, violations are less likely to be detected under an HMO system than under fee-for-service programs. Moreover, the guidelines must not require the curtailment of services that physicians believe to be essential, lest doctors provide such services and invent fraudulent ways to bill for them.

AN INTERNATIONAL
PERSPECTIVE

International surveys repeatedly show Americans to be less satisfied with their medical system than residents of other countries. In a poll conducted simultaneously in the United States, Canada, and Britain in 1989, for example, only 10 percent of the Americans said their health care system functioned "pretty well," compared with 56 percent of Canadians and 27 percent of British respondents. Far more Americans than Canadians or British said financial barriers kept them from getting the health care they needed, and 89 percent of the Americans believed the nation's health care system required fundamental change.[49]

Americans were also significantly less satisfied than the Canadians and the British with their last visit to a physician. Only 54 percent of the Americans said they were "very satisfied" with that visit, compared to 63 percent of the British and 73 percent of Canadians. Sixty-one percent of the Americans said they preferred the Canadian system of health care; only 3 percent of the Canadians and 12 percent of the British preferred the American system.[50]

The following brief survey of three foreign national health systems highlights the relationship between structural arrangements, quality of care, and fraud. Beyond structural variations, we may note, the way medicine is practiced differs notably from country to country and plays into the amount and detection of fraud. International differences in medical practice are more significant than the similarities, according to a recent survey conducted by Lynn Payer. She noted, for instance, that the prescribed dose of a drug varied among the four countries she surveyed—the United States, England, West Germany, and France—by as much as tenfold and twentyfold, though there is little difference in the mortality rates within the countries. French patients have a seven times greater chance of getting suppositories than Americans. Blood pressure deemed high enough for treatment in the United States is considered normal in England. Low blood pressure, believed to be desirable by American doctors, is treated in West Germany. In France, only 2.4 percent of all women have hysterectomies; in the United States, 2 percent of women between thirty-five and forty-four have hysterectomies each year.[51]

Great Britain

In 1982 the New Times Gallup Hospital Market Research group found that only 16 percent of the Americans surveyed preferred a medical system like that of England. British citizens, however, strongly support their national health program and do not want to change it, though they would like to see the system upgraded by the infusion of additional funds; two-thirds said they were willing to pay more taxes to improve it.[52] The *Washington Post* may have been guilty of hyperbole when it maintained that the program is "revered" in England, but the contrast between public approval in England for the National Health Service (NHS) and public dissatisfaction in the United States is striking.

Recent attempts by conservatives in the British government to reduce the NHS budget by privatizing some of its segments drew a barrage of criticism. The most succinct critique was given by David Owen, a physician and at the time an opposition party leader: "The commercialization of health care is the primrose path down which inexorably lies American medicine: first-rate treatment for the wealthy and tenth-rate treatment for the poor."[53]

The NHS, with about one million employees, is believed to be Europe's largest single employer. Doctors earn about $50,000 annually from the program, and some supplement their government earnings by seeing private patients.[54] The leading complaint against the British program concerns the long waits for nonemergency surgeries. At the beginning of 1989, the list for elective surgery included 660,000 persons. Partly because of this situation, about 5.3 million of Britain's 57 million residents carry private medical insurance.[55]

The British have also openly adopted controversial social considerations in decisions about the deployment of medical resources—issues that have not yet been confronted on a national scale in the United States. For example, in Britain, younger persons are given preference for kidney dialysis; patients over fifty-five might or might not be accorded such treatment, and those over seventy-five never receive it. The absence of financial incentives for performing complex procedures also reduces the prevalence of such procedures. Since British surgeons are salaried and not paid by the case, for example, they have no financial temptation to operate when it is not necessary. In part because of this, coronary bypasses are performed ten times more often in the United States than in Britain, though there is no evidence that heart disease kills earlier or more often in Britain than in this country.

Britain spends only 5.5 percent of its gross national product on medical care, less than any other industrialized nation, and administrative costs are only 4 percent of the health care budget, compared to 20 percent of all health care expenditures in the United States.[56] (The claim that the British health service is bankrupting the country is undercut by Britain's recent budget surplus, as compared to America's multibillion dollar deficits.) Despite the differences in costs, the British people appear as healthy as their American counterparts or more so. One study found that on seventeen measures of health, the British people were fourth among the ten nations surveyed, though their country spent less than any of the others on medical care. The United States was second in spending but ninth in health. Another rating scale, measuring the ability of countries to provide for their people, found the United States ranked behind most Western European countries.[57]

The government's move into health care in Britain, as in the United States, produced a significant increase in the demand for services. But in Britain the increased demand effected only a small rise in medical costs, while American costs soared. The key difference, according to one analyst, has been "the effectiveness of third-party controls (especially control by the central government) over spending."[58]

The NHS does not publish statistics about violations of the system by physicians. However, the tactic of restricting the number of patients any NHS doctor can have on his or her panel seems to be an effective method for monitoring and deterring fraud, because it regularizes the extent of any one practice and makes statistical deviations in treatment procedures stand out sharply. At times, senior consultant physicians do drag their feet in dealing with NHS patients, subtly suggesting they would get faster treatment if they returned as private patients. But this self-serving behavior seems to be isolated. Overall, the British system is far less susceptible to fraud and abuse than a fee-for-service system.[59]

Canada

Most commentators believe the Canadian medical care system offers the best blueprint for national health insurance in the United States. Uwe Reinhardt, a leading authority on medical programs in the United States, concluded, "If I were a physician who really cared about patients, I'd probably prefer the Canadian system." The *New England Journal of Medicine* reported early in 1989 that Physicians for a National Health Program, a group of twelve hundred American doctors, supported a change to the Canadian system, noting that "our health care system is failing." Dissenting voices, however, insist a Canadian-style program would not work in the United States because the population is too geographically dispersed for effective administration and because the United States cannot match Canada's history of excellence in state-run services.[60]

The Canadian system, called Medicare, began to take its present form in 1962, when the province of Saskatchewan introduced universal public coverage of all medical expenses. By 1971 all the provinces had inaugurated Medicare programs. Canadian Medicare is a fully government-funded insurance program that sets doctors' and hospitals' fees; nearly 90 percent of Canada's 40,000 doctors participate in the program. Patients are free to select their own doctors and hospitals. Canadian hospitals have few machines to blast away kidney stones, but no woman who wants prenatal care goes unattended.[61]

In 1971, when Canada's national program started, Canada and the United States each spent about 7.5 percent of their gross national product on health. While Canada has held that proportion to 8 percent, the U.S. figure has risen to 12 percent.[62] Part of the differential in health costs reflects doctors' fees. Canadian doctors, a 1990 report indicated, charge only half of what U.S. doctors charge. The annual income of U.S. doctors is only about one-third more than that of Canadian doctors, however, because the latter see more patients.[63]

Though doctors remain Canada's best-paid professionals, they have been restive at times regarding their incomes. In 1982 Quebec's general practitioners staged a labor slowdown that included rotating walkouts and refusals to treat nonemergency patients. After five days, the government forced the doctors to return to work. Over the years, some Canadian physicians have left for the United States in search of higher incomes.

Little official attention at the federal level has been paid to the question of fraud in Canada's Medicare, because the provinces are assumed to exert stringent control. Canadian authorities suggest that the scarcity of private hospitals, which account for about 70 percent of U.S. inpatient services, is a strong curb on fraud and abuse. Nonetheless, in Australia, where fewer than one in three hospitals is private, fraud is regarded as widespread.[64]

The Canadian Medical Association (CMA) maintains that its emphasis on high ethical standards and its careful monitoring of doctors' work have effectively deterred violations. An alternative hypothesis, however, posits that the CMA has been particularly successful in diverting attention from "what invariably is a painful and sometimes a costly matter for the medical fraternity."[65] The Canadian public's relative indifference to Medicare fraud seems largely to be the result of Canadian physicians' dominance over the enforcement process. In British Columbia, for instance, Medicare forwards information on deviant practices to the British Columbia Medical Association's Patterns of Practice Committee, a body designated to determine whether practitioners are billing incorrectly or providing medically unnecessary services. A majority of the committee is appointed by the medical association itself; thus the profession retains a sure grip on which cases are investigated. No charge has ever been successfully laid in British Columbia for fraud or other abuses of the medical program. Instances of fraud documented by independent analysts were defined by the profession as "mistakes" and "misunderstandings" rather than criminal behavior.[66]

The experience of Quebec, however, was quite different. During its first three years of operation, Quebec's Health Insurance Board prosecuted sixty cases and produced thirty convictions. There were more prosecutions in Quebec than in all other Canadian provinces combined. That physicians in Quebec were less honest than their colleagues in other provinces is implausible. The difference, rather, resided in the enforcement procedures: Quebec's Health Insurance Board "chose to deal directly with these cases rather than by a peer review approach."[67] Quebec's board uses computer programs to identify physicians whose practices deviate from the statistical norms, and those doctors are summoned before the board. In Quebec, it has been common for the board to require a deviating doctor to undertake a particular course of postgraduate study or have a second consultant in all subsequent cases of certain diagnoses.[68]

Australia

Australia adopted its present system of national health care in 1965, after an intense battle between politicians and organized medicine.[69] "No profession has resisted inroads into its power better," one writer remarks apropos the struggle and its aftermath.[70] The fee-for-service system provides medical benefits to all Australian residents and generally covers 85 percent of a practitioner's scheduled fees. In 1984 a 1 percent income tax surcharge was enacted to help finance the program.

Careful studies of "medifraud"—the Australian term for it—have focused on three phenomena that create conditions conducive to criminal behavior: the structure of organized medicine; the socialization and training of student physicians; and the economics of the medical marketplace, which is distorted by an oversupply of physicians.[71]

Enforcement efforts are said to be seriously hampered by inadequate staff resources in the Fraud and Overservicing Detection Scheme (FODS) and by bureaucratic difficulties in coordinating investigative inquiries. In addition, the Australians are said to take a kid-glove approach to doctors, preferring to counsel those engaged in overservicing rather than to take punitive action. This opinion is borne out by a comprehensive scholarly analysis of medifraud prosecution and sentencing between 1975 and 1982. In that period, only fifty-one doctors were prosecuted—fewer than ten a year. The conviction rate was 84 percent, with slightly more than half (55 percent) of all the convictions resulting in fines and about 30 percent resulting in orders to pay restitution. Four physicians received prison terms. One was released after a month; the remaining eleven months of the sentence were suspended when the doctor filed a good behavior bond. Two doctors received three-year prison terms, with a minimum release date set at nine months, and the fourth doctor received an eight-month sentence. In sum, relatively few doctors are prosecuted for medifraud and the penalties imposed are relatively light.[72]

Peter Cashman, who conducted the analysis of medifraud, observes that the frauds "are very hard to investigate," the legislation is badly drafted, and "in order to establish the extent of the offense it is necessary to bring a large number of charges in respect to all of the claims made." On this last point an Australian solicitor concurs, noting that unless each fraud is documented, the amount involved would be "so piddling that you'd be laughed out of court."[73]

A person familiar with fraud prosecutions of Australian physicians notes:

Given that the penalty imposed rarely, if ever, reflects the extent of the suspected fraud, the doctor is not discouraged from abuse of the system. Indeed, his experience in court will have acquainted him with the probable consequences so that he will only become more devious and clever in his future abuse of the system. Such doctors are literally in the position of "laughing all the way to the bank," for they know that even if they are caught again, the gains far exceed any penalties.[74]

These remarks seem to us considerably overstated. Few people, even if fraud proves financially profitable, will amiably undergo the experience of being a defendant in a criminal procedure. What the quotation reflects more fundamentally is the same cynical attitude in this Australian observer that we find so often in Americans familiar with the rip-offs that take place in the Medicaid program.

Late in 1977 an officer of the Medibank Private company examined an American report on medical fraud and, on the basis of its findings and his own investigations, prepared an estimate of fraud in Australia. When his superior rejected the report, he left the company and shared his information with the media. Despite sporadic media attention, though, Australian politicians ignored medical fraud until 1982, when it became a continuing issue of national concern:

With the advent of the Medibank Mark I computerized information system, it became possible to draw a reasonably accurate picture of an individual doctor's practice. It soon became apparent that some doctors' workloads were markedly different from those of most of their peers. Clearly a significant degree of overservicing was occurring, and some doctors' claims for payment of social service beneficiaries were fraudulent. . . . Senior spokesmen of the AMA [Australian Medical Association] admitted that deception on a large scale had been practiced by some doctors. It has been suggested that 10 percent or more of total payments of medical services per year may have been claimed fraudulently.[75]

By one estimate, pathology is among the subspecialties yielding the highest losses through fraud. Fraud by pathologists is almost impossible to prove, however. After the initial tests are ordered by the referring doctor, Australian pathologists retain the right to order any further tests they believe necessary. No analyses are conducted in the presence of patients, so there is no opportunity for even rudimentary patient monitoring.[76]

General Observations

Despite basic structural differences, there are important similarities in the medical programs in Australia, Canada, and the United States.

First, in all three countries physicians are reimbursed on a fee-for-service basis. Second, in each case the major medical associations lobbied against universal national health insurance. Third, doctors rank as the highest-paid professional group in their respective countries. Finally, each health care system is currently under attack, both by physicians and by budgetary constraints. In recent years, Australia's labor government has been offering the medical profession concessions believed to weaken the National Health Scheme.[77] In Canada doctors are pressing for "user charges" (fees above reimbursements from Medicare) and permission to "extra bill," that is, to charge patients small amounts in addition to what the government will pay. The analogous problems of Medicare and Medicaid in the United States need not be repeated here.

All three countries report difficulties in securing resources for policing medical fraud. The intricacies of criminal law requirements and problems in persuading prosecutors to bring charges are also common complaints among enforcement officials in each of the countries. The dollar amount of an alleged fraud is said to be crucial in determining whether an investigation or a prosecution is undertaken.

In all three countries, despite different traditions and approaches to health care, the common forms of medical fraud and abuse seemed similar enough for one research team to suggest similar susceptibility of all fee-for-service benefit programs to standardized criminal acts.[78] To a great extent, the nature of medical benefit program crimes may be conditioned by the nature of health care delivery as it has evolved in contemporary industrialized capitalist societies. When doctors retain strong control over their billing practices, some are going to be tempted to bilk the system.

Unfortunately, data are not available on fraud and abuse in European health programs that do not adhere to a fee-for-service approach. Perhaps the matter is of little consequence because such fraud might have been infrequent. In Eastern Europe, at least before the 1989 and 1990 upheavals and probably still today, medicine was rife with practices regarded as wholly unprofessional elsewhere. In the Soviet Union, a "shadow medical economy" had come into existence. Influence and gifts were employed to obtain appointments with hard-to-see specialists, and state doctors were often bribed to see patients after hours. Nurses demanded favors such as flowers, candy, or liquor to give basic hospital care to patients. Such practices were so common that people considered them part of everyday life.[79]

In Britain, as we have seen, doctors are salaried and their patient load is controlled. The salaried status of doctors in hospitals, one analyst concluded, "removes any financial involvement for [physicians] and so they have no incentive to 'overprovide' services." The British system also respects doctors' professional autonomy: "A salary and a consultant status [allow] hospital doctors in the NHS a great deal of freedom to do their work as they wish."[80] But the structural pitfall here (as we said earlier of HMOs in the United States) might be undertreatment.

As we have noted, no one has yet devised a method for determining the actual extent of medical fraud in the United States. Nor is there a satisfactory method for determining whether the extent of medical fraud in Canada or Australia matches or exceeds the estimated U.S. rates. The level of overall crime is significantly lower in these other countries than in the United States, and the ethos of law-abidingness may also extend to medical practitioners. But in the United States, Australia, and Canada, cheating by doctors is regarded as a significant problem that is not readily amenable to solution, particularly because of the power of the medical societies.

WHERE ARE WE GOING?

The American public believes that all Americans, regardless of income, deserve quality medical care and that the current system is a miserable failure on this score. In January 1990 President George Bush designated his secretary of health and human services to lead a Domestic Policy Council review of recommendations on the quality, accessibility, and cost of the nation's health care system. But his brief comments on this appointment emphasized the need "to bring the staggering costs of health care under control." The economic figures bore out his concern: From 1988 to 1989, the cost of employers' medical plans jumped by 20.4 percent, and Medicaid program expenditures rose by 12 percent.[81]

A reporter for the *New York Times* interpreted Bush's announcement to signify that "universal health care has been elevated to a Presidential matter." Secretary Louis Sullivan promised to undertake "an overview of the entire system . . . to develop real improvements and to control costs."[82] To date, the Bush administration has done little.

Two months after Bush's speech, the Bipartisan Commission on Comprehensive Health Care (the Pepper Commission) issued a set of recommendations. The commission urged the states and the federal government to require companies having more than a hundred employees to provide their work force with medical insurance. The commission also advocated that a publicly funded plan be established to cover the medical expenses of all persons without private insurance. The estimated first-year cost of the latter proposal was $66 billion, about the same amount attached to a similar proposal advocated by the AMA, which hoped to ensure federal funding for medical bills while also ensuring that "the patients' freedom to choose their health-care provider" remained inviolate.[83] The cost of these proposals, however, seems prohibitive, especially given that the proposed federal budget called for an $800 million cut in federal Medicaid funding for fiscal year 1990–91.

A radically different approach to cost containment is under way in Oregon's Medicaid program. The state appointed an eleven-person panel to review 1,600 medical procedures and to devise a cost-benefit formula that balanced the price tag for a procedure against the severity of the patient's illness and the benefit of the treatment. The state's goal was to be able to afford to increase the number of poor persons eligible for Medicaid by rationing expensive services and refusing to pay for some procedures. Controversy arose after disclosure of the initial rankings revealed that crooked teeth were near the top of the priority list, while bone and liver transplants as well as treatment of AIDS patients nearing death were toward the bottom.[84] Oregon cannot afford to finance the program without its share of federal Medicaid funds, and the Bush administration has been unwilling to bend existing Medicaid rules to allow funding of the experiment.

Meanwhile, public opinion surveys continue to testify to declining satisfaction with the current system. In a nationwide poll conducted by the *Los Angeles Times* in February 1990, for instance, more than half the 2,046 respondents indicated that the entire American health care system needed "many improvements" or "fundamental overhauling" and that they would be willing to pay additional taxes for reform. Sixty-nine percent believed that medical costs could be "substantially reduced" without affecting the quality of health care. A similar majority said the government should take the lead both in controlling costs and improving coverage and access to care. Seventy-two percent of the respondents favored national health insurance, and two-thirds of respondents favored the Canadian system of health care delivery. Health care ranked fifth among the most frequently identified problems facing the country, behind drug abuse, crime, the federal deficit, and the economy.

Doctors, too, were dissatisfied with the state of medicine, according to a front-page story in the *New York Times* on February 18, 1990:

Dramatic changes in medical practice have shattered the profession, leaving many doctors deeply demoralized.

Over the past quarter-century, and especially in the last 10 years, doctors have seen their autonomy eroded, their future earning potential jeopardized, their prestige reduced and their competence challenged by everyone from oversight boards to hostile, litigious patients.

The image of the dedicated physician toiling long hours for the good of his patients is fading fast, replaced by salaried doctors who work 9 to 5.[85]

One sign of the growing pressure for physician accountability was an announcement by Johns Hopkins Hospital that it would begin testing doctors for drug and alcohol use—the first testing program in an acute-care or community hospital. There was, assuredly, a certain calculated shrewdness underlying the Hopkins policy. For one thing, the testing of physicians was to be carried out only every two years. For another, the tactic was the apparent forerunner of a program to test nurses and other employees whose participation obviously could more readily be enlisted if the doctors were not exempt. The hospital's vice-president noted that the program's sponsors were "very eager this not be punitive." The AMA thought the move "an interesting experiment."[86]

At the same time, the dismemberment of Medicaid continues apace. In August 1989 the nation's governors asked the president and the Congress to impose a two-year moratorium on additional mandated

Medicaid benefits because Medicaid was growing faster than any other state program, rising from 10 percent of state budgets in 1985 to 14 percent in 1990, with a projected increase to 17 percent in 1995.

To control costs, seven states—Arkansas, Florida, Kansas, Massachusetts, Tennessee, Vermont, and Washington—had enacted limits on doctors' visits. In Massachusetts and Florida, Medicaid recipients are deterred from consulting several physicians for the same ailment by a program limit of one doctor visit a day. In Vermont, the limit is five visits a month. In Kansas, some recipients, depending on the services they receive, are restricted to twelve to twenty-four visits a year. But more stringent restrictions were imposed by New York State—with a Medicaid enrollment of 2.3 million persons—in 1989. These "utilization thresholds" permit fourteen nonemergency visits annually and eighteen laboratory tests, though emergency rooms must treat all patients and the ceiling can be lifted if a doctor certifies that a patient needs extra care. Doctors and hospitals, claiming that the certification procedure would be "arduous," presumed that the net result would be that some needy people would go untreated. Other restrictions pertain to dental work, podiatry, and drugs.

These restrictions were expected to save New York State about $50 million a year in its current $11 billion Medicaid budget. Although the state has the highest number of Medicaid convictions in the nation, it nonetheless loses more money to fraud than any other state. Auditors there have to cope with nine million Medicaid claims each month.[87] Meanwhile, Medicaid fraud continues apace. Among the larger frauds, by dollar value, was that perpetrated by the owner of three clinical laboratories. In 1987 his medical license was revoked for Medicaid fraud. In 1989 he pled guilty to cheating Medicaid of $3.6 million by buying huge quantities of human blood from drug addicts and other ill or poor people and then running unordered and unnecessary tests on it. He purchased the blood for about $10 a vial, and each pint of blood yielded as much as $2,000 in billings for tests. The defrocked doctor's laboratories had accounted for more than 20 percent of Medicaid billings from the state's 450 laboratories.[88]

A New York City physician earned a million dollars a year and a reputation as the "Dwight Gooden of Medicaid billers"—for having "an arm that won't quit," in the words of a fraud investigator. Patients lined up at the sixty-one-year-old physician's storefront office at 5 A.M. and waited hours for a half-minute examination. The doctor almost invariably handed them a prescription for $150 or more worth of drugs. A typical "examination" was witnessed by a reporter. An unemployed thirty-two-year-old patient said he had come to the office because of problems with alcohol and a variety of pains.

> "So?" asked the doctor. "You are doing better. You are not drinking?"
> "Oh, yes, doctor," said the patient. "Thanks to you."
> "Your life is better than before?"
> "Yes."

With that, the doctor signed a prescription for two-week to one-month supplies of Buspar, a tranquilizer; Zantac, an ulcer medication; Elavil, an antidepressant; Proventil, an inhaler used to quell asthmatic symptoms; Feldene, an anti-inflammatory drug that eases back pain; and Lotrimin, a cream for rashes. (The patients generally sold the drugs or used some to supplement their hard-drug habits.) In discussing this case, the state's special Medicaid fraud prosecutor underlined "the ever-present difficulty of proving criminal bad faith beyond a reasonable doubt, particularly in those cases where at least some minimum physical examination has been performed."[89]

Over the years, various proposals have been made for measures to reduce Medicare and Medicaid fraud: increase the reimbursement rates, emphasize ethics and social responsibility in school curriculums and required refresher courses, increase enforcement efforts, establish punishments that involve shaming, [90] eliminate the fee-for-service structure. Certainly, it is time for the government to reconsider the assumptions that the architects of the federal benefit program took for granted. As Federal District Judge Charles L. Bricant, Jr., of New York, explained:

Those greater minds than ours who contrived this Medicaid legislation created a very easy and obvious means to steal public funds. Why did they do this? I think the answer is twofold.

First, legislators thought that physicians were above that sort of thing because of the education they have, because of the respect they received from the community, and because of the standing they have, that they would not do any such thing.

I think also that the government believed they did not want bureaucrats intervening between the physician and his patients solely to prevent fraud. Their expectations were not fulfilled.[91]

Crimes by physicians against Medicaid, like all crimes in the United States, seem to occur at an unconscionably high rate. We seem no closer than we ever have been to controlling the level of such degradations as rape, murder, and robbery. Maybe, like these terrors, Medicaid fraud is yet another perverse offspring of a social system that drives its communicants to try to achieve specified cultural goals for themselves but that fails to convey an adequate understanding that this achievement is to be sought only within the confines of the legally permissible. Crime will be reduced in the United States only when people no longer desire, are not able to get at, or are afraid to try to secure those kinds of things that, either by nature or by experience, they have come to want. Manipulation of any of these elements in the acquisitive equation—desire, opportunity, or the fear of consequences—would help bring Medicaid fraud under better control. That something must—and very likely will—be done about the problem seems evident from the material we have gathered regarding the form and the extent of the abuse of the Medicaid program by physicians. Whether such change will help the health of poor patients remains open to debate.

As we saw in chapter 1, enforcement of the laws regarding drugs and abortions led the white, male-dominated medical profession to abandon certain types of patients. To date, the enforcement of Medicaid rules and regulations has had a similar effect. When Medicaid was enacted, legislators believed that most doctors would see some Medicaid patients. But perceived needless paperwork and bureaucratic control have dissuaded the majority of physicians from participating in the program, so that poor patients have been left to seek health care from a limited number of doctors. Increased policing will probably exacerbate the situation. The lesson from other countries seems to be that this dilemma can be solved only by structural changes in the delivery of health care in the United States.

Notes

Chapter 1

1. Ellen Hume, "The AMA Is Laboring to Regain Dominance over Nation's Doctors," *Wall Street Journal*, 13 June 1986.

2. Patricia McCormack, "Once Hospital Board Insider: Carter Reveals Taking Part in Medical 'Ripping Off,'" *Los Angeles Times*, 25 Apr. 1979.

3. E. Richard Brown, *Rockefeller Medicine Men: Medicine and Capitalism in America* (Berkeley: University of California Press, 1979), 82.

4. Jonathan Gathrone-Hardy, *Doctors: The Lives and Work of GPs* (London: Corgi Books, 1987), 155.

5. Morris J. Vogel, *The Invention of the Modern Hospital, Boston, 1870–1930* (Chicago: University of Chicago Press, 1980), 2; Brown, *Rockefeller Medicine Men*, 99.

6. Vogel, *Invention of the Modern Hospital*.

7. Brown, *Rockefeller Medicine Men*.

8. John Espar, "A Physicians' Market," honors thesis, Indiana University, 1984.

9. Sylvia A. Law, *Blue Cross: What Went Wrong?* (New Haven: Yale University Press, 1974).

10. Robert D. Eilers, "The Fundamental Nature of Blue Cross and Blue Shield," *Journal of Insurance* 12 (1962): 35.

11. Robert D. Eilers, *Regulation of Blue Cross and Blue Shield Plans* (Homewood, Ill.: Richard D. Irwin, 1963).

12. Ibid., 16.

13. Robert Pear, "Physicians Contend Systems of Payment Have Eroded

Status," *New York Times*, 26 Dec. 1987; Dirk Johnson, "Doctors' Dilemma: Unionizing," *New York Times*, 13 July 1987.

14. Glenn Ruffenach, "No Need to Worry, Doctors Do Just Fine," *Wall Street Journal*, 10 Oct. 1988; Hume, "The AMA"; "Physicians' Incomes in Sharp Rise," *Orange County Register*, 21 Oct. 1987.

15. Milt Freudenheim, "Medical Costs Continue to Surge: Evasion of Controls Held a Cause," *New York Times*, 20 July 1986.

16. Phil Keisling, "Radical Surgery: Let's Draft the Doctors," *Washington Monthly* 14 (1983): 26–34, quote at 30.

17. Norman Cousins, *Anatomy of an Illness as Perceived by the Patient: Reflections on Healing and Regeneration* (New York: Norton, 1979), 137–38.

18. Pear, "Physicians"; Sonja Steptoe, "Hassles and Red Tape Destroy Joy of the Job for Many Physicians," *Wall Street Journal*, 20 Apr. 1987; Samuel Garth, *The Dispensary, A Poem*, 12th ed. (Dublin: George Risk, 1697/1730).

19. Paul Marcotte, "MD Salaries Rise Again—Easily Surpassing Lawyers," *American Bar Association Journal* 74 (1988): 17.

20. Tom Goldstein, "No Straight A's for the Law Schools," *New York Times*, 10 Jan. 1988.

21. David Margolick, "Lawyers' Bilked Clients Getting Day in Court," *Orange County Register*, 5 Jan. 1988.

22. Stephen M. Rosoff, "Physicians as Criminal Defendants: Specialty Status and Sanctions," doctoral dissertation, University of California, Irvine, 1987; G. Counts, "The Social Status of Occupations: A Problem in Vocational Guidance," *School Review* 33 (1925): 16–27; John Alfred Nietz, "The Depression and the Social Status of Occupations," *Elementary School Journal* 16 (1935): 575–86; M. E. Deeg and D. G. Paterson, "Changes in Social Status of Occupations," *Occupations* 25 (1947): 205–6; C. W. Hall, "Social Prestige Values of a Selected Group of Occupations," *Psychological Bulletin* 35 (1938): 696–99; G. Hartman, "The Prestige of Occupations," *Personnel Journal* 13 (1934): 144–52; Charles Osgood and Ross Stagner, "Analysis of a Prestige Frame of Reference by a Gradient Technique," *Journal of Applied Psychology* 25 (1941): 275–90; Richard Simpson and Ida Simpson, "Correlates and Estimates of Occupational Prestige,"*American Journal of Sociology* 66 (1960): 135–40; Maryon K. Welsh, "The Ranking of Occupations on the Basis of Social Status," *Occupations* 27 (1949): 237–41.

23. National Opinion Research Center, "Jobs and Occupations: A Popular Evaluation," *Opinion News* 9 (1941): 3–13; Gene I. Maeroff, "Polls Say

Americans Support Raises and Tests for Teachers," *New York Times*, 2 July 1985.

24. Rosoff, "Physicians as Criminal Defendants"; Louis Harris and Associates, *Medical Practice in the 1980's: Physicians Look at Their Changing Profession* (Menlo Park, Calif.: Kaiser Foundation, 1981); Perri Klass, *A Not Entirely Benign Procedure: Four Years as a Medical Student* (New York: Putnam, 1987).

25. Harvey Cushing, *The Life of Sir William Osler* (London: Oxford University Press, 1940), 447, 177.

26. Select Committee on Aging, U.S. House of Representatives, *Medicare: A Fifteen-Year Perspective* (Washington, D.C.: U.S. Government Printing Office, 1980).

27. Committee on Finance, U.S. Senate, *Medicare-Medicaid Fraud and Abuse Amendments of 1977* (Washington, D.C.: U.S. Government Printing Office, 1977).

28. Pawel Horoszowski, *Economic Special-Opportunity Conduct and Crime* (Lexington, Mass.: Lexington Books, 1978), 151.

29. Al Messerschmidt, "Witnesses Dispute Doctor's Claims," *Miami Herald*, 16 Jan. 1982; Shula Beyer, "Doctor Gets Twenty Years for Medicaid Fraud," *Miami Herald*, 6 Mar. 1982; Fred Grimm, "Woman Doctor Convicted in Plot to Kill Partner Sentenced to Life," *Miami Herald*, 4 Feb. 1983.

30. Peter Kihss, "Medicaid Fraud Laid to Carriers," *New York Times*, 26 Sept. 1971; Donald C. Bacon, "Medicaid Abuse: Even Worse Than Feared," *U.S. News and World Report*, 4 June 1979, 43–45.

31. Emile Durkheim, *Le Suicide: Etude de Sociologie* (Paris: Felix Alcan, 1897), 53.

32. Horoszowski, *Economic Conduct and Crime*.

33. Talcott Parsons, *The Social System* (Glencoe, Ill.: Free Press, 1951), 435.

34. Ibid., 472–73.

35. Anthony Weinlein, "Pharmacy as a Profession with Special Reference to the State of Wisconsin," master's thesis, University of Chicago, 1943; Isador Thorner, "Pharmacy: The Functional Significance of an Institutional Pattern," *Social Forces* 20 (1942): 321–28.

36. Richard Quinney, "Occupational Structure and Criminal Behavior: Prescription Violations by Retail Pharmacists," *Social Problems* 11 (1963): 179–85.

37. Ibid., 181, 183–84.

38. John Braithwaite, "White-Collar Crime," *Annual Review of Sociology* 11 (1985): 1–25.

39. Edwin H. Sutherland, "White-Collar Criminality," *American Sociological Review* 5 (1940): 1–12.

40. Edwin H. Sutherland, *White-Collar Crime* (New Haven: Yale University Press, 1983), 7; originally published 1949.

41. Ibid., 1, and Sutherland's unpublished notes; see also Robert S. Myers, "The Rise and Fall of Fee-Splitting," *Bulletin of the American College of Surgeons* 40 (1955): 507–9, 523; Howard Whitman, "Why Some Doctors Should Be in Jail," *Collier's* 132 (1953): 23–27.

42. Selig Greenberg, *The Quality of Mercy* (New York: Atheneum, 1978).

43. Lonn Lanza-Kaduce, "Deviance Among Professionals: The Case of Unnecessary Surgery," *Deviant Behavior* 1 (1980): 333–59.

44. Richard D. Lyons, "Surgery on Poor Is Found Higher," *New York Times*, 1 Sept. 1977.

45. Constance M. Winslow et al., "The Appropriateness of Performing Coronary Artery Bypass Surgery," *Journal of the American Medical Association* 260 (1988): 505–9; Alain Enthoven, "A 'Cost-Conscious' Medical System," *New York Times*, 13 July 1989.

46. Alan L. Otten, "How Medical Advances Often Worsen Illnesses and Even Cause Death," *Wall Street Journal*, 27 July 1988.

47. Robert Welkos, "Doctor Involved in Blindings Is Given a 4-Year Term for Fraud," *Los Angeles Times*, 27 Apr. 1984.

48. John Bunker and John Wennberg, "Operation Rates, Mortality Statistics, and the Quality of Life," *New England Journal of Medicine* 289 (1973): 1249–51.

49. Howard H. Hiatt, "Protecting the Medical Commons: Who Is Responsible?" *New England Journal of Medicine* 293 (1975): 241–93.

50. Harry J. Anslinger and Will Oursler, *The Murderers! The Shocking Story of the Narcotic Gangs* (New York: Farrar, Straus, and Cudahy, 1961).

51. David S. Musto, *The American Disease: Origins of Narcotic Control* (New Haven: Yale University Press, 1973), 121.

52. Ibid., 123, 132; Alfred R. Lindesmith, *The Addict and the Law* (Bloomington: Indiana University Press, 1965).

53. Richard Gordon, *A Question of Guilt: The Case of Dr. Crippen* (New York: Atheneum, 1981); Sybille Bedford, *The Best We Can Do: An Account of the Trial of John Bodkin Adams* (London: Collins, 1958); Patrick Devlin, *Easing the Passing: The Trial of Dr. John Bodkin Adams* (London: Collins,

1985); Percy Hoskins, *Two Men Were Acquitted: The Trial and Acquittal of Dr. John Bodkin Adams* (London: Secker and Warburg, 1984); Cesare Lombroso, *Crime: Its Causes and Remedies*, trans. Henry P. Horton (Boston: Little, Brown, 1911), 58.

54. Paul Goldstein, *Prostitution and Drugs* (Lexington, Mass.: Lexington Books, 1982), 43.

55. Mike Goodman and George Reasons, "Law Cripples Probe of Medi-Cal Fraud," *Los Angeles Times*, 23 Mar. 1978.

56. Barbara Katz Rothman, *Recreating Motherhood: Ideology and Technology in a Patriarchal Society* (New York: Norton, 1989).

57. Kristin Luker, *Abortion and the Politics of Motherhood* (Berkeley: University of California Press, 1984).

58. James C. Mohr, *Abortion in America: The Origins and Evolution of National Policy, 1800–1900* (New York: Oxford University Press, 1978), 163, 164.

59. Ibid., 164.

60. Lucy Freeman, *The Abortionist* (Garden City, N.Y.: Doubleday, 1962); Nancy Howell Lee, *The Search for an Abortionist* (Chicago: University of Chicago Press, 1969).

61. Jerome E. Bates and Edward S. Zawadzki, *Criminal Abortion: A Study in Medical Sociology* (Springfield, Ill.: Thomas, 1964), 3.

62. Frederick J. Taussig, *Abortion Spontaneous and Induced: Medical and Social Aspects* (St. Louis: Mosby, 1936), 422.

63. Bates and Zawadzki, *Criminal Abortion*, 36.

64. Jacqueline D. Forrest, Ellen Sullivan, and Christopher Tietze, "Abortion in the United States, 1976–1977," *Family Planning Perspectives* 10 (1978): 271.

65. Jonathan B. Imber, *Abortion and the Private Practice of Medicine* (New Haven: Yale University Press, 1986), 77, 119.

66. John Keown, *Abortion, Doctors and the Law: Some Aspects of the Legal Regulation of Abortions in England from 1803 to 1982* (Cambridge: Cambridge University Press, 1986), 40, 46.

67. *Rex v. Bourne*, 3 All Eng. Reports 615 (1938).

68. Keown, *Abortion*, 87, 159.

69. Howard S. Becker and Blanche Geer, "The Fate of Idealism in Medical School," *American Sociological Review* 23 (1958): 50.

70. Robert K. Merton, George C. Reader, and Patricia L. Kendall, eds., *The Student Physician* (Cambridge: Harvard University Press, 1957), 77–78.

71. Leonard D. Eron, "The Effect of Medical Education on Attitudes: A Follow-Up Study," *Journal of Medical Education* 33 (1958): 25–33; Louise B. Miller and Edmond F. Erwin, "A Study of Attitudes and Anxiety in Medical Students," *Journal of Medical Education* 34 (1959): 1089; Leonard V. Gordon and Ivan N. Mensh, "Values of Medical Students at Different Levels of Training," *Journal of Educational Psychology* 53 (1962): 48–51; R. Gray and W. R. Newman, "The Relationship of Medical Students' Attitudes of Cynicism and Humanitarianism to Performance in Medical School," *Journal of Health and Human Behavior* 3 (1962): 147–51.

72. Miller and Erwin, "Attitudes and Anxiety in Medical Students"; George Saslow, "Psychiatric Problems in Medical Students," *Journal of Medical Education* 31 (1956): 27–33; Caroline Bedell Thomas, "What Becomes of Medical Students: The Dark Side," *Johns Hopkins Medical Journal* 138 (1976): 185–95; Carol C. Nadelson, Malkah T. Notman, and David W. Preven, "Medical Student Stress, Adaptation and Mental Health," in *The Impaired Physician*, ed. Stephen C. Scheiber and Brian B. Doyle (New York: Plenum, 1983); David Langsley, foreword to *The Impaired Physician*, ix.

73. Paul Jacobs, "Future Doctors: Are Schools Screening Out the Best?" *Los Angeles Times*, 11 Feb. 1953.

74. Donald R. Cressey, *Other People's Money: The Social Psychology of Embezzlement* (New York: Free Press, 1953), 16–20.

75. James H. Price et al., "Perceptions of Family Practice Residents Regarding Health Care and Poor Patients," *Journal of Family Practice* 27 (1988): 615–21.

76. Everett C. Hughes, "The Making of a Physician—General Statement of Ideas and Problems," *Human Organization* 14 (1956): 23.

77. Michael Medved, *Hospital: The Hidden Lives of a Medical Center Staff* (New York: Simon and Schuster, 1982), 239.

78. Becker and Geer, "The Fate of Idealism," 50–56.

79. Samuel W. Bloom, *Power and Dissent in the Medical School* (New York: Free Press, 1973); Merton, Reader, and Kendall, *The Student Physician*; Virginia L. Olesen and Elvi W. Whittaker, *The Silent Dialogue: A Study in the Psychology of Professional Socialization* (San Francisco: Jossey-Bass, 1968).

80. Jack Haas and William Shaffir, "The Professionalization of Medical Students: Developing Competence and a Cloak of Competence," *Symbolic Interaction* 1 (1977): 73.

81. Haas and Shaffir, "Professionalization," 71–72 and passim.

82. Carol Klaperman Morrow, "The Medicalization of Professional Mis-

conduct," paper presented at the meeting of the American Sociological Association, Toronto, 1981.

83. Haas and Shaffir, "Professionalization," 73.

84. Eliot Freidson, *Doctoring Together: A Study of Professional Social Control* (New York: Elsevier, 1975).

85. Parsons, *The Social System.*

86. Margot Jeffreys and Mary Ann Elston, "The Medical School as a Social Organization," *Medical Education* 23 (1989): 242–51.

87. Lawrence P. Levitt, "The Personality of the Medical Student: A Brief Historical Review and Contemporary Psychiatric Study," *Chicago Medical School Quarterly* 25 (1966): 201–14; R. C. Hunter, R. H. Prence, and A. E. Schwartzman, "Comments on the Emotional Disturbances in a Medical Undergraduate Population," *Canadian Medical Association Journal* 85 (1961): 989–92; Stephen C. Scheiber, "The Medical School Admissions Committee: A Preventive Psychiatry Challenge," in *The Impaired Physician*, ed. Scheiber and Doyle.

88. Peter MacGarr Rabinowitz, *Talking Medicine: America's Doctors Tell Their Stories* (New York: New American Library, Mentor Books, 1983), 60.

89. David G. Johnson, *Physicians in the Making* (San Francisco: Jossey-Bass, 1983), 37–38; Brown, *Rockefeller Medicine Men.*

90. Erwin O. Smigel, "Public Attitudes Toward Stealing as Related to the Size of the Victim Organization," *American Sociological Review* 21 (1956): 320–27.

91. Jeffreys and Elston, "The Medical School as a Social Organization," 245.

92. Steven C. Martin, Ruth M. Parker, and Robert M. Arnold, "Careers of Women Physicians: Choices and Constraints," *Western Journal of Medicine* 149 (1988): 759.

93. Constance Keenan et al., "Medical Students' Attitudes on Physician Fraud and Abuse in the Medicare and Medicaid Programs," *Journal of Medical Education* 60 (1985): 167–73.

94. David Matza, *Delinquency and Drift* (New York: Wiley, 1964), 28–29.

95. Ibid., 42.

Chapter 2

1. Quoted in Subcommittee on Long-Term Care, Special Committee on Aging, U.S. Senate, *Fraud and Abuse Among Practitioners Participating in*

the Medicaid Program (Washington, D.C.: U.S. Government Printing Office, 1976), 84.

2. Ibid.

3. Ibid.

4. Stuart Auerbach, "31 Area Doctors Hold Drug Repackaging Stock," *Washington Post,* 11 Aug. 1966; Alice Bonner, "U.S. to Crack Down on Medicaid Fraud," *Los Angeles Times,* 27 Mar. 1976.

5. "Medical Overcharges Up to 400% Reported," *Los Angeles Times,* 27 July 1976; Subcommittee on Long-Term Care, *Fraud and Abuse,* 1; "More Medicaid Fraud Disclosed by Panel, but Quick Remedies in Congress Unlikely," *Wall Street Journal,* 31 Aug. 1976.

6. Frank Campion, *The AMA and U.S. Health Policy Since* 1940 (Chicago: Chicago Review Press, 1984), 154.

7. Campion, *The AMA;* Richard Arnold and David Eisenstadt, "The Effects of Medical Society Control of Blue Shield on Fees in the Physician Service Market: Some Preliminary Evidence," *Quarterly Review of Economics and Business* 22 (1982): 31–44; Harry Schwartz, "Doctors Debate How to Split the Fees," *Wall Street Journal,* 15 Jan. 1985.

8. Lewis E. Weeks and Howard J. Berman, *Shapers of U.S. Health Policy: An Oral History* (Ann Arbor, Mich.: Health Administration Press, 1985), 63; Campion, *The AMA.*

9. "The Big Push," *New England Journal of Medicine* 265 (1961): 1317; Campion, *The AMA.*

10. Kenneth R. Wing, "The Impact of Reagan-Era Politics on the Federal Medicaid Program," *Catholic University Law Review* 33 (1983): 93; Austin C. Wehrwein, "New Health Plan Offered by A.M.A.," *New York Times,* 10 Jan. 1965; Weeks and Berman, *Shapers of U.S. Health Policy,* 73; Campion, *The AMA,* 275; Robert Stevens and Rosemary Stevens, *Welfare Medicine in America: A Case Study of Medicaid* (New York: Free Press, 1974).

11. Jennifer O'Sullivan, "Medicaid: Fiscal Year 1982 Administrative Budget Proposal," Library of Congress Congressional Research Service (Mini Brief MB81231), 1981.

12. Karen Davis and Cathy Schoen, *Health and the War on Poverty: A Ten-Year Appraisal* (Washington, D.C.: Brookings Institution, 1978), 18.

13. Philip J. Hilts, "U.S. Reports Drop in Infant Deaths," *New York Times,* 6 Apr. 1991; "U.S. Health Gap Is Getting Wider," *New York Times,* 23 Mar. 1990.

14. U.S. House of Representatives, "Medicare Gaps and Limitations: Hearing Before the Subcommittee on Health and Long-Term Care of the Select Committee on Aging," 18 Oct. 1977.

15. Title II, U.S.C., Section 208.

16. Elliot Freidson, *Professional Dominance: The Social Structure of Medical Care* (New York: Atherton, 1970); Stephen Chapman, "More Cost-Sharing Needed to Avert a Medicare Crisis," *Orange County Register*, 17 Jan. 1984.

17. Campion, *The AMA*, 256.

18. Theodore Marmor, *Politics of Medicare* (Chicago: Aldine, 1973), 80.

19. Weeks and Berman, *Shapers of U.S. Policy*, 93.

20. Stevens and Stevens, *Welfare Medicine*, 132.

21. Ibid., 264.

22. Subcommittee on Long-Term Care, *Fraud and Abuse*, 87.

23. Eric Malnic, "Pharmacist Given Prison Term for Medi-Cal Claims," *Los Angeles Times*, 9 Mar. 1968.

24. Committee on Finance, U.S. Senate, *Medicare and Medicaid: Hearings* (Washington, D.C.: U.S. Government Printing Office, 1969); Richard Lyons, "Medicare Study in Senate Seeks Urgent Reforms," *New York Times*, 9 Feb. 1970.

25. Committee on Finance, U.S. Senate, *Medicare and Medicaid: Hearings Before Subcommittee on Medicare-Medicaid* (Washington, D.C.: U.S. Government Printing Office, 1970).

26. Subcommittee on Long-Term Care, *Fraud and Abuse*.

27. Jay Nelson Tuck, "Medicaid: Why the Program Is Mortally Ill," *New York Times*, about 1969; Nancy Hicks, "Medicaid Fee Abuse Report Attacked," *New York Times*, 11 Feb. 1970.

28. Robert McFadden, "'Medical Cop' for City," *New York Times*, 27 Sept. 1971.

29. Pater Kihss, "Medicaid Fraud Laid to Carriers," *New York Times*, 26 Sept. 1971.

30. Quoted in Subcommittee on Long-Term Care, *Fraud and Abuse*, 90.

31. Ibid., 91.

32. Ibid., 93.

33. Edward Ranzal, "Kickbacks Found on Health Tests," *New York Times*, 11 Jan. 1973; M. A. Farber, "State to Study Medicaid Fraud," *New York Times*, 8 Feb. 1973.

34. Stuart L. Auerbach, "Medicaid Examiners Cite Fraud Findings," *Los Angeles Times*, 30 Aug. 1976.

35. Subcommittee on Long-Term Care, *Fraud and Abuse*, 26.

36. Auerbach, "Medicaid Examiners."

37. John Hess, "New York Officials Place Medicaid Frauds at 20%," *New York Times*, 31 Aug. 1976.

38. George Vecsey, "Dr. Matthew Calls Arrest 'A Political Thing' by D.A.," *New York Times*, 2 Apr. 1973.

39. Ibid.; Paul Delaney, "'All Assistance Possible' to Matthew Reported Ordered Personally by Nixon," *New York Times*, 11 Dec. 1973.

40. Lawrence Van Gelden, "Interfaith Loses Certificate Bid," *New York Times*, 1 May 1973.

41. Barbara Campbell, "Matthew Says Diverted Funds from Medicaid Aided Patients," *New York Times*, 19 Oct. 1973; John Sibley, "Matthew Guilty in Medicaid Fraud," *New York Times*, 8 Nov. 1973.

42. Sibley, "Matthew Guilty"; Mary Breasted, "Pressure Is Cited in Matthew Case," *New York Times*, 29 Nov. 1973; Linda Charlton, "S.B.A. Aide Says He Refused to Destroy Audit on Matthew," *New York Times*, 1 Dec. 1973.

43. Gary Granville, "Cella: King-Turned-Con Toils Quietly," *Orange County Register*, 1982.

44. Jack Katz, "Legality and Equality: Plea Bargaining in the Prosecution of White-Collar and Common Crimes," *Law and Society Review* 13 (1979): 431–59.

45. "U.S. Medicaid Audit Finds 90% Errors," *Los Angeles Times*, 11 Feb. 1977; "U.S. Lists the Doctors Convicted for Frauds in Medicare-Medicaid," *New York Times*, 1 June 1979.

46. Helen Smits, "PSROs: Origins, Directions, and Changing Assumptions," *Bulletin of the New York Academy of Medicine* 58 (1982): 11–18.

47. Campion, *The AMA*, 330; Barry Decker and Paul Bonner, *PSRO: Organization for Regional Peer Review* (Cambridge, Mass.: Ballinger, 1973), 6–7.

48. Feather A. Davis, "The Evaluation of Professional Standards Review Organizations: Their Part in the Struggle to Assure Appropriate Health Care," *Bulletin of the New York Academy of Medicine* 58 (1982): 67–76.

49. Fred Richardson, "Peer Review of Medical Care," *Medical Care* (Jan.–Feb. 1972): 1; Freidson, *Professional Dominance*; Edward N. Peters, "Practical Versus Impractical Peer Review," *Medical Care* 10(Nov.–Dec. 1972): 516–21.

50. Lawrence D. Brown, "Political Conditions of Regulatory Effectiveness:

The Case of PSROs and HSHs," *Bulletin of the New York Academy of Medicine* 58 (1982): 77–90, quote at 78–79.

51. Claudia Wallis, "Weeding Out the Incompetents," *Time*, 26 May 1986, 57–58.

52. Committee on Finance and Special Committee on Aging, U.S. Senate, *Oversight of HHS Inspector General's Effort to Combat Fraud, Waste, and Abuse* (Washington, D.C.: U.S. Government Printing Office, 1982), 2.

53. Harvey F. Pies, "Control of Fraud and Abuse in Medicare and Medicaid," *American Journal of Law and Medicine* 3 (1977): 323–32, quote at 328.

54. Elizabeth E. Hogue, Sanford V. Teplitzky, and Howard L. Sollins, *Preventing Fraud and Abuse: A Guide for Medicare and Medicaid Providers* (Owings Mills, Md.: National Health Publishing, 1988), 2.

55. Ibid., 3.

56. "State Investigative Unit Orders Jailing of a Witness at Inquiry into Medicaid," *New York Times*, 25 June 1975; "Medicaid Inquiry on Coast Finds Kickbacks and Bribes," *New York Times*, 19 Mar. 1980.

57. Committee on Finance and Special Committee on Aging, *Oversight*.

58. Richard P. Kusserow, *Semi-Annual Report (April–September), Office of Inspector General* (Washington, D.C.: U.S. Government Printing Office, 1989); U.S. Comptroller General, *Federal Funding for State Medicaid Fraud Control Units Still Needed: Report to Congress* (Washington, D.C.: General Accounting Office, 1980).

59. Select Committee on Aging, U.S. House of Representatives, *Medicaid Fraud: A Case History in the Failure of State Enforcement* (Washington, D.C.: U.S. Government Printing Office, 1982), 59.

60. Harry Nelson, "Transfer of the 'Medically Needy' Stirs Apprehension," *Los Angeles Times*, 3 Oct. 1982.

61. David Johnston, "Medi-Cal Panel Created to Redraw 'Medical Monster,'" *Los Angeles Times*, 8 Nov. 1979.

62. Robert Fairbanks and Carl Ingram, "Legislature OKs 1st Step in Shakeup of Health Care," *Los Angeles Times*, 25 June 1982; Nelson, "Transfer."

63. Larry Peterson, "New Strategy Devised to Trim $200 Million from Medi-Cal Plan," *Orange County Register*, 9 July 1982; Charles Petit, "Harshest in 16 Years: The Effect of Medi-Cal Cutbacks," *Los Angeles Times*, 2 Sept. 1982.

64. Nicole Lurie et al., "Termination from Medi-Cal—Does It Affect Health?" *New England Journal of Medicine* 311 (1984): 480–84.

65. Bob Egelko, "Medi-Cal Must Give Notice of Benefit Cuts," *Orange County Register,* 2 Sept. 1989.

66. Michael Waldholz, "New Views About Care in Hospitals Lead to Slower Rise in Health Costs," *Wall Street Journal,* 8 Oct. 1984.

67. Michael J. Zimmerman, *An Essay on Human Action* (New York: P. Lang, 1984), 48–55.

68. Hogue, Teplitzky, and Sollins, *Preventing Fraud.*

69. Wallis, "Weeding Out the Incompetents," 57–58.

70. Sharon McIlrath, "PRO Sanction Boom Matches MD Resentment," *American Medical News,* 2 Jan. 1987.

71. Mark Rust, "Justice Says Peer Review Not an Antitrust Violation," *American Medical News,* 19 Dec. 1986.

72. Sharon McIlrath, "PRO Contract Negotiations Under Way Soon," *American Medical News,* 11 Mar. 1988.

73. Frank Thompson, *Health Policy and the Bureaucracy: Politics and Implementation* (Cambridge: MIT Press, 1983), 153.

74. Stuart C. Hadden and Marilyne Lester, "Looking at Society's Troubles, the Sociology of Social Problems," in *Understanding Social Problems,* ed. Don H. Zimmerman, Laurence D. Wieder, and Sin Zimmerman (New York: Praeger, 1976), 11. See also Herbert Blumer, "Social Problems as Collective Behavior," *Social Problems* 18 (1971): 298–306.

75. John Gardiner and Theodore Lyman, *Fraud Control Game* (Bloomington: Indiana University Press, 1981), 4.

Chapter 3

1. John Braithwaite, *To Punish or Persuade: Enforcement of Coal Mine Safety* (Albany: State University of New York Press, 1985).

2. "U.S. Medicaid Audit Finds 90% Errors," *Los Angeles Times,* 11 Feb. 1977.

3. Martin Bulmer, "The Research Ethics of Pseudo-Patient Studies: A New Look at the Merits of Covert Ethnographic Methods," *Sociological Review* 30 (1982): 627–46.

4. "U.S. Bares Gouge by Medics," *New York Times,* 2 June 1961.

5. Jack Katz, "Legality and Equality: Plea Bargaining in the Prosecution of White-Collar and Common Crimes," *Law and Society Review* 13 (1979):

431; Select Committee on Aging, U.S. House of Representatives, *Medicaid Fraud: A Case History in the Failure of State Enforcement* (Washington, D.C.: U.S. Government Printing Office, 1982), 33.

6. Alan Stone, "The Legal Implications of Sexual Activity Between Psychiatrist and Patient," *American Journal of Psychiatry* 133 (1976): 1138–41.

7. Michael Crichton, *Travels* (New York: Random House, 1988), 62–63.

8. Austin Scott, "Medicaid Expert Subpoenaed after Defying Order to Testify," *Washington Post*, 1 Oct. 1976.

9. Select Committee on Aging, *Medicaid Fraud*, 66.

10. Orrin Hatch, testimony, Committee on Labor and Human Resources, U.S. Senate, 10 July 1984, 4–15.

11. Arnold Rosoff, testimony, Committee on Labor and Human Resources, U.S. Senate, 10 July 1984, 25–40.

12. Hatch, testimony, 5.

13. Joel Brinkley, "A.M.A. Study Finds Big Rise in Claims for Malpractice," *New York Times*, 17 Jan. 1985.

14. Keith Hawkins, *Environment and Enforcement: Regulation and the Social Definition of Pollution* (Oxford: Clarendon Press, 1983).

15. Donald J. Black, "The Social Organization of Arrest," *Stanford Law Review* 23 (1971): 733.

16. Select Committee on Aging, *Medicaid Fraud*.

17. Jell Weir, "OC Doctor to Undergo Sanity Trial," *Orange County Register*, 15 May 1984.

18. Dave Patermo, "Investigators Contend Use of 'Drivers' to Solicit Patients Key to Scheme," *Los Angeles Times*, 25 Aug. 1985.

19. M. Pham, open letter (unpublished), 1984.

20. *People v. Barazza*, 23 Cal. 3d 675, 153 Cal. Rptr. 459, 591 P.2d 104 (1979).

21. John Braithwaite, Brent Fisse, and Gilbert Geis, "Covert Facilitation and Crime: Restoring Balance to the Entrapment Debate," *Journal of Social Issues* 43 (1987): 5.

22. Marshall B. Clinard and Peter C. Yeager, *Corporate Crime* (New York: Macmillan, 1980).

23. *Sherman v. Sherman*, Root 486 (Conn. 1793); Alan Westin, *Privacy and Freedom* (New York: Atheneum, 1967), 325.

24. Dina Khajezadeh, "Patient Confidentiality Statutes in Medicare and Medicaid Fraud Investigations," *American Journal of Law and Medicine* 13 (1987): 105–37.

25. *Commonwealth v. Kobrin*, No. SJC 3671, Supreme Judicial Court, Commonwealth of Massachusetts (1985).

26. Doug Smith, "Providers Are Hard to Catch, Fraud Division Finds," *Arkansas Gazette*, 18 Apr. 1982.

27. Edwin Sutherland, *White-Collar Crime* (New Haven: Yale University Press, 1983), 251–52; originally published 1949.

28. John T. Noonan, *Bribes* (New York: Macmillan, 1984).

29. Vicki Ong, "Medicaid Problem: Not Aware of 'Big Fraud,'" *Honolulu Advertiser*, 27 June 1985; "Fraud Unit Review," *Mini News*, 26 June 1985; Ken Kobayashi, "Medicaid Fraud Chief," *Honolulu Advertiser*, 7 Aug. 1985.

30. Johannes Andenaes, "Deterrence and Specific Offenses," *University of Chicago Law Review* 38 (1971): 537; Frank Zimring and Gordon Hawkins, *Deterrence: The Legal Threat in Crime Control* (Chicago: University of Chicago Press, 1973).

31. Henry M. Pontell, *A Capacity to Punish* (Bloomington: Indiana University Press, 1984).

32. Richard Kusserow, "Civil Money Penalties Law of 1981: A New Effort to Confront Fraud and Abuse in Federal Health Care Programs," *Notre Dame Law Review* 58 (1983): 985–94.

33. *Trop v. Dulles*, 356 U.S. 86 (1958); *Chapman v. U.S.*, 521 F.2d 523 (1987).

34. James Q. Wilson, *Bureaucracy: What Government Agencies Do and Why They Do It* (New York: Basic Books, 1989), 174; Jack Katz, *Seductions of Crime: Moral and Sensual Attractions in Doing Evil* (New York: Basic Books, 1988), 318.

35. Theodore R. Marmor, *The Politics of Medicare* (Chicago: Aldine, 1970), 15.

36. Barry R. Furrow et al., *Health Law: Cases, Materials and Problems* (St. Paul: West, 1987); T. Buchberger, *Medicaid: Choices for 1982 and Beyond* (Washington, D.C.: Congressional Budget Office, Congress of the United States, 1981).

37. "Medicaid Acceptance: A Problem in Pennsylvania," *American Medical News*, 3 July 1987.

38. Michael W. Jones and Bette Hamburger, "A Survey of Physician Participation in and Dissatisfaction with the Medi-Cal Program," *Western Journal of Medicine* 124 (1976): 75–83.

Chapter 4

1. Subcommittee on Long-Term Care, Special Committee on Aging, U.S. Senate, *Fraud and Abuse Among Practitioners Participating in the Medicaid Program* (Washington, D.C.: U.S. Government Printing Office, 1976), 81.

2. Committee on Finance and Special Committee on Aging, U.S. Senate, *Oversight of HHS Inspector General's Effort to Combat Fraud, Waste, and Abuse* (Washington, D.C.: U.S. Government Printing Office, 1982), 34–40, quote at 36.

3. Ronald Sullivan, "Health Chief for New York to Act Against Misconduct by Physicians," *New York Times*, 3 Apr. 1983.

4. Nanette Gartrell et al., "Psychiatrist-Patient Sexual Contact: Results of a National Survey, I: Prevalence," *American Journal of Psychiatry* 143 (Sept. 1986): 1126–31.

5. Edward Alsworth Ross, "The Criminaloids," *Atlantic Monthly* 99 (1907): 44–50.

6. Stanton Wheeler, Kenneth Mann, and Austin Sarat, *Sitting in Judgment: The Sentencing of White-Collar Criminals* (New Haven: Yale University Press, 1988), 155.

Chapter 5

1. Gresham Sykes and David Matza, "Techniques of Neutralization: A Theory of Delinquency," *American Sociological Review* 22 (1957): 664–70.

2. Donald Cressey, *Other People's Money: A Study in the Social Psychology of Embezzlement* (New York: Free Press, 1953).

3. David Matza, *Delinquency and Drift* (New York: Wiley, 1964).

4. Sykes and Matza, "Techniques of Neutralization," 667.

5. Ibid.

6. Ibid., 668.

7. Ibid.

8. Ibid.

9. Theodor Adorno et al., *The Authoritarian Personality* (New York: Harper, 1950).

10. Sykes and Matza, "Techniques of Neutralization," 669.

11. Matza, *Delinquency and Drift*, 33, 59.

12. Johannes Andenaes, "General Prevention Revisited: Research and Policy Implications," *Journal of Criminal Law and Criminology* 66 (1975): 338–65.

Chapter 6

1. Emile Durkheim, *Suicide: A Study in Sociology*, trans. John A. Spaulding and George Simpson (New York: Free Press, 1951), 254; original French ed. published 1897.

2. Talcott Parsons, *The Social System* (Glencoe, Ill.: Free Press, 1951).

3. Arnold S. Relman, "Doctors and the Dispensing of Drugs," *New England Journal of Medicine* 317 (1987): 311.

4. Parsons, *The Social System*.

5. Paul Starr, *The Social Transformation of Medicine* (New York: Basic Books, 1982), 360, 427.

6. Parsons, *The Social System*, 468.

7. Joseph Ripple, Letter to the Editor, *Wall Street Journal*, 14 Aug. 1987.

8. David E. Hyde, "Who Says There's a Physician Surplus?" *American Medical News*, 16 Jan. 1987.

9. Alain Enthoven, "A 'Cost-Conscious' Medical System," *New York Times*, 13 July 1989; Uwe E. Reinhardt, "The U.S. System: Errors of Youth," *Washington Post*, 15 Mar. 1988.

10. Art Buchwald, "Why the Malady Lingers On," *Los Angeles Times*, 12 Apr. 1983.

11. Hubert Wallot and Jean Lambert, "Characteristics of Physician Addicts," *American Journal of Drug and Alcohol Abuse* 10 (1984): 53–62; William E. McAuliffe, "Nontherapeutic Opiate Addiction in Health Professionals: A New Form of Impairment," *American Journal of Drug and Alcohol Abuse* 10 (1984): 1–22; Kenneth N. Vogtsberger, "Treatment Outcomes of Substance-Abusing Physicians," *American Journal of Drug and Alcohol Abuse* 10 (1984): 23–37; G. E. Vaillant, J. R. Brighton, and C. McArthur, "Physicians' Use of Mood-Altering Drugs: A Twenty-Year Follow-up Report," *New England Journal of Medicine* 282 (1970): 365–70; H. C. Modlin and A. Montes, "Narcotic Addiction in Physicians," *American Journal of Psychiatry* 121 (1964): 358–65; William E. McAuliffe et al., "Psychoactive Drug Use by Young and Future Physicians," *Journal of Health and Social Behavior* 25 (1984): 34–54.

12. Robert S. Walzer, "Impaired Physicians: An Overview and Update of the Legal Issues," *Journal of Legal Medicine* 11 (1990): 131–98; Wallot and

Lambert, "Characteristics of Physician Addicts," 220, 61; McAuliffe, "Nontherapeutic Opiate Addiction"; McAuliffe et al., "Psychoactive Drug Use."

13. J. G. Bruhn and O. A. Parsons, "Medical Student Attitudes Towards Four Medical Specialities," *Journal of Medical Education* 30 (1964): 40–49; J. Hammond and F. Hern, *Teaching Comprehensive Medical Care* (Cambridge: Harvard University Press, 1959); D. G. Wilkinson, S. Greer, and B. K. Toone, "Medical Students' Attitudes to Psychiatry," *Psychological Medicine* 13 (1983): 185–92.

14. Donald Light, *Becoming Psychiatrists: The Professional Transformation of Self* (New York: Norton, 1980), 24, 42.

15. Andrew Scull, *Decarceration* (Englewood Cliffs, N.J.: Prentice-Hall, 1976).

16. Brian B. Doyle and David W. Cline, "Approaches to Prevention in Medical Education," in *The Impaired Physician*, ed. Stephen C. Scheiber and Brian B. Doyle (New York: Plenum, 1983), 51–68.

17. Deborah Allen, "Women in Medical Specialty Societies: An Update," *Journal of the American Medical Association* 262 (1989): 3439–43; Kathryn McGoldrick, "Gender and Economics," *Journal of the American Medical Women's Association* 43 (1988): 103.

18. Freda Adler, *Sisters in Crime: The Rise of the New Female Criminal* (New York: McGraw-Hill, 1975).

19. Rita James Simon, *The Contemporary Woman and Crime* (Washington, D.C.: U.S. Government Printing Office, 1975), 48.

20. Meda Chesney-Lind, "Women and Crime: The Female Offender," *Signs: Journal of Women in Culture and Society* 12 (1986): 78–96; Kenneth Tardiff, "A Model for Short-Term Prediction of Violence Potential," in *Current Approaches to the Prediction of Violence*, ed. David A. Brizer and Martha Crowner (Washington, D.C.: American Psychiatric Association, 1989).

21. Carol Gilligan, *In a Different Voice* (Cambridge: Harvard University Press, 1982); on men and women in the workplace, Michael Betz and Lenahan O'Connell, "Gender and Work: A Look at Sex Differences Among Pharmacy Students," *American Journal of Pharmaceutical Education* 51 (1987): 39–43; on workplace ruses, Richard Blum, *Surveillance of Espionage in a Free Society* (New York: Praeger, 1982); on medical students, Jane Leserman, *Men and Women in Medical School: How They Change and How They Compare* (New York: Praeger, 1981), 198.

22. Ruth Martin, *Witchcraft and the Inquisition in Venice, 1550–1650* (Oxford: Basil Blackwell, 1989), 226.

23. Starr, *Social Transformation of Medicine,* 391.

24. Steven C. Martin, Robert M. Arnold, and Ruth M. Parker, "Gender and Medical Specialization," *Journal of Health and Social Behavior* 29 (1988): 333–43; Allen, "Women in Medical Specialty Societies"; Angela Holder, "Women Physicians and Malpractice Suits," *Journal of the American Medical Women's Association* 34 (1979): 239–40.

25. Ferris N. Pitts, Jr., et al., "Suicide Among U.S. Women Physicians," *American Journal of Psychiatry* 13 (1979): 696.

26. Joel Best and David F. Luckenbill, "Male Dominance and Female Criminality: A Test of Harris's Theory of Deviant Type-Scripts," *Sociological Inquiry* 60 (1990): 71–86; Judith Lorber, *Women Physicians: Careers, Status, and Power* (New York: Tavistock, 1984).

27. Janet Mitchell, "Medicaid Participation by Medical and Surgical Specialties," *Medical Care* 12 (1983): 929.

28. On specialties, see Allen, "Women in Medical Specialty Societies"; on self-employment, see Martin, Arnold, and Parker, "Gender and Medical Specialization."

29. Kathleen Daly, "Gender and Varieties of White-Collar Crime," *Criminology* 27 (1989): 769–93; Dorothy Zietz, *Women Who Embezzle or Defraud: A Study of Convicted Felons* (New York: Praeger, 1981); Clair M. Callan and Eve Klipstein, "Women Physicians in Connecticut: A Survey," *Connecticut Medicine* 45 (1981): 494–96; Marcia Angell, "Women in Medicine: Beyond Prejudice," *New England Journal of Medicine* 304 (1981): 1161–63; Marilyn Heins et al., "Productivity of Women Physicians," *Journal of the American Medical Association* 236 (1976): 1961–64; Eleanor Nash, "Depression in Medical Women," *Journal of the American Medical Women's Association* 43 (1988): 176–80; LeClair Bissel and Jane K. Skorina, "One Hundred Alcoholic Women in Medicine," *Journal of the American Medical Association* 267 (1987): 2939–44; Gabrielle A. Carlson and Diane C. Miller, "Suicide, Affective Disorder, and Women Physicians," *American Journal of Psychiatry* 138 (1981): 1330–35; Martina S. Horner, "Toward an Understanding of Achievement-Related Conflicts in Women," *Journal of Social Issues* 28 (1972): 157–75; Alexandra Symonds, "Emotional Conflicts and Career Women: Women in Medicine," *American Journal of Psychoanalysis* 43 (1983): 21–37.

30. Gilbert Geis and Robley Huston, "Trends in the Dismissal of Tenured Teachers," in *The Yearbook of School Law,* ed. Lee O. Garber (Danville, Ill.: Interstate Publishers, 1962).

31. Margaret Engel, "Doctors Said to Be Laxly Monitored," *Washington*

Post, 1 Sept. 1985; Ronald Sullivan, "Doctors Submit to Drug Tests as Alternative to Penalties," *New York Times*, 13 Mar. 1987; Carol K. Morrow, "Sick Doctors: The Social Construction of Professional Deviance," *Social Problems* 30 (1982): 92–108.

32. Margaret Engel, "Medical Tests Revamped to End Cheating," *Washington Post*, 27 Apr. 1985; John Carlova, "How Many Doctors Are Cheating Their Way into Practice?" *Medical Economics*, 6 Feb. 1984, 84–92; Marian Sandmaier, "Doctor No: When M.D. Spells Trouble," *Mademoiselle*, Mar. 1987, 174–84.

33. Carlova, "How Many Doctors Are Cheating?" 87; Joel Brinkley, "28,000 'Doctors' Are Feared Unfit," *New York Times*, 5 May 1986.

34. "Bad Doctors," *Public Citizen* 10 (1990): 6.

35. Charlotte L. Rosenberg, "How Bad Doctors Dodge Discipline," *Medical Economics*, 18 Mar. 1985, 211–219.

36. Ibid.; Joel Brinkley, "Crossing the State Lines Can Offer Haven for Dangerous Doctors," *Louisville Courier-Journal*, 8 Aug. 1982.

37. Margaret Engel, "One in Five Military Doctors Lacks License," *Washington Post*, 10 July 1987.

38. Edwin Chen, "Data Banks on Physicians," *Los Angeles Times*, 28 Nov. 1989; Philip J. Hilts, "Oversight, Phase I: Keeping Records of Doctors with Records," *New York Times*, 9 Sept. 1990.

39. Engel, "Doctors Said to Be Laxly Monitored."

40. Daniel Ein, "Malpractice Insurance: A Search for Solutions," *Washington Post*, 24 Feb. 1986.

41. Greg Easterbrook, "The Revolution in Medicine," *Newsweek*, 26 Jan. 1987, 40–74.

42. Eugene G. McCarthy, Madston Lubin Finkel, and Hirsh S. Ruchlin, *Second Opinion Elective Surgery* (Boston: Auburn House, 1981), ii.

43. Starr, *Social Transformation of Medicine*, 392.

44. Ibid., 445, 448.

45. George Ritzer, "Sociology at Work: A Metatheoretical Analysis," *Social Forces* 67 (1989): 593–600.

46. Allan Parrachini, "Health Care Debate: Who Will Pay the Way?" *Los Angeles Times*, 30 Aug. 1987.

47. Reinhardt, "The U.S. System"; Dennis Hevesi, "Poll Shows Discontent with Health Care," *New York Times*, 15 Feb. 1989.

48. Allan Parrachini, "Doctors Differ in Need for Health Care," *Los Angeles Times*, 10 June 1984.

49. Hevesi, "Polls Show Discontent with Health Care."

50. Ibid.

51. Lynn Payer, *Medicine and Culture: Varieties of Treatment in the United States, England, West Germany, and France* (New York: Henry Holt, 1988), 24–25.

52. Parrachini, "Health Care Debate"; Jonathan Randal, "Thatcher Unveils Health Care Reform," *Washington Post*, 1 Feb. 1989.

53. Steve Lohr, "Free-Market Health System: New Thatcher Goal for Britain," *New York Times*, 1 Feb. 1989.

54. Karen De Young, "The British Love Their National Health Service: But Can It Survive?" *Washington Post*, 15 Mar. 1988.

55. Lohr, "Free-Market Health System"; Craig R. Whitney, "Thatcher's New Health Plan: An Outcry Rises on All Sides," *New York Times*, 26 June 1989.

56. Ripple, Letter to the Editor.

57. For the first study, see Barry Newman, "Socialized Care: Frugal Medical Service Keeps Britons Healthy and Patiently Waiting," *Wall Street Journal*, 9 Feb. 1983; for the second, see Richard J. Estes, *Trends in World Social Development: The Social Progress of Nations, 1980–1986* (New York: Praeger, 1988), 105–7.

58. J. Rogers Hollingsworth, *A Political Economy of Medicine: Great Britain and the United States* (Baltimore: Johns Hopkins University Press, 1980), 135.

59. Milton I. Roemer, *Comparative National Policies on Health Care* (New York: Marcel Dekker, 1977), and telephone interview, 22 Mar. 1991.

60. Reinhardt, "The U.S. System"; David V. Himmelstein and Steffie Woolhandler, "A National Health Program for the United States," *New England Journal of Medicine* 320 (1989): 102–8; Henry M. Lerner, "Don't Look to Canada's Health System," *New York Times*, 3 Feb. 1990.

61. Malcolm G. Taylor, *Health Insurance and Canadian Public Policy*, 2d ed. (Kingston: McGill-Queen's University Press, 1987); Robert G. Evans, *Strained Mercy: The Economics of Canadian Health Care* (Toronto: Butterworth's, 1984); Elisabeth Rosenthal, "In Canada, a Government System That Provides Health Care to All," *New York Times*, 30 Apr. 1991.

62. Victor R. Fuchs, "How Does Canada Do It? A Comparison of Expenditures for Physicians' Services in the United States and Canada," *New England Journal of Medicine* 323 (1990): 884–90.

63. Ibid.

64. Liaison Committee, "Medical Fraud," *Journal of Solicitor-Generals Department* (Ottawa: Government Printer, 1985), 25; Joint Committee on Public Accounts, *Minutes of Evidence: Medical Fraud and Overservicing*, vols. 1–9 (Canberra: Australian Government Publishing Service, 1982), 63; *Medical Fraud and Overservicing*, Report 203 (Canberra: Australian Government Publishing Service, 1984), 3.

65. Paul Wilson and Pam Gorring, "Social Antecedents of Medical Fraud and Overservicing: What Makes a Doctor Criminal," *Australian Journal of Social Issues* 20 (1985): 175–87.

66. Charles Ennals, "Winds of Change in Patterns of Practice," *British Columbia Medical Journal* 26 (1984): 31–35; Paul Wilson, Duncan Chappell, and Robyn Lincoln, "Policing Physician Abuse in British Columbia: An Analysis of Current Policies," *Canadian Public Policy* 12 (1986): 236–44; Wilson and Gorring, "Social Antecedents of Medical Fraud"; Paul Wilson, Duncan Chappell, and Robyn Lincoln, "Physician Fraud and Abuse in Canada: A Preliminary Examination," *Canadian Journal of Criminology* 28 (1986): 129–46.

67. Gordon Hatcher, *Universal Free Health Care in Canada, 1944–1977* (Washington, D.C.: U.S. Government Printing Office, 1981), 138.

68. Roemer, *Comparative National Policies*, 178.

69. James A. Gillespie, *The Price of Health: Australian Governments and Medical Politics* (New York: Cambridge University Press, 1990).

70. L. J. Opit, "Wheeling, Healing and Dealing: The Political Economy of Health Care in Australia," *Community Health Studies* 7 (1983): 238–46, 233.

71. Paul Wilson, "Medical Fraud and Abuse in Medical Benefit Programmes," in *Stains on a White Collar: Fourteen Studies in Corporate Crime or Corporate Harm*, ed. Peter Grabosky and Adam Sutton (Annandale, Australia: Foundation Press, 1989), 76, 81.

72. Peter Cashman, "Medical Benefit Fraud: Prosecution and Sentencing of Doctors," *Legal Services Bulletin* 7 (1982): 58–61 (Part I), 116–21 (Part II).

73. Ibid., Part I, 59.

74. Ibid., Part II, 119.

75. John Dewdney, "Health Services in Australia," in *Comparative Health Systems: Descriptive Analyses of Fourteen National Health Systems*, ed. Marshall W. Raaffel (University Park: Pennsylvania State University Press, 1983), 43.

76. Wilson, "Medical Fraud and Abuse."

77. John A. Gardiner and Theodore R. Lyman, *The Fraud Control Game: State Responses to Fraud and Abuse* (Bloomington: Indiana University Press, 1984); Dewdney, "Health Services in Australia," 9; Wilson and Gorring, "Social Antecedents of Medical Fraud."

78. Paul Wilson, Gilbert Geis, Henry N. Pontell, Paul Jesilow, and Duncan Chappell, "Medical Fraud and Abuse: Australia, Canada, and the United States," *International Journal of Comparative and Applied Criminal Justice* 9 (1985): 25–34.

79. Esther B. Fein, "More and More in Private Soviet Medical Clinics, the Doctor Is Out," *New York Times*, 5 Mar. 1989.

80. David Allen, "Health Services in England," in *Comparative Health Systems*, 243.

81. "Medical Plan Costs Rise 20.4% in '89, Study Shows," *Wall Street Journal*, 30 Jan. 1990; Milt Freudenheim, "Cutting the Cost of Medicaid Drugs," *New York Times*, 30 Jan. 1990.

82. Hilts, "Oversight, Phase I."

83. Robert A. Rosenblatt, "Divided Panel Presents $66 Billion Medical-Care Plan," *Los Angeles Times*, 3 Mar. 1990; "AMA Urges Medicaid Changes to Improve Nation's Health Care," *Orange County Register*, 8 Mar. 1990.

84. "Nation's First Medicaid-Rationing Program Falls Behind Schedule," *Orange County Register*, 20 Aug. 1990.

85. Lawrence Altman and Elisabeth Rosenthal, "Changes in Medicine Bring Pain to Healing Profession," *New York Times*, 18 Feb. 1990.

86. Tamar Levin, "Johns Hopkins to Institute Drug Tests on Physicians," *New York Times*, 10 Feb. 1990.

87. Sam Howe Verhovek, "New York to Limit Medicaid Services to 2.3 Million People to Control Costs," *New York Times*, 16 Aug. 1989, and "New York State Move to Curb 'Medicaid Mills' Draws Criticism," *New York Times*, 30 Sept. 1989.

88. Craig Wolff, "Medicaid Bilking Is Admitted," *New York Times*, 14 Mar. 1989.

89. Sam Howe Verhovek, "Doctor Who Billed Millions Is Cut by N.Y. Medicaid," *New York Times*, 6 Nov. 1989.

90. John Braithwaite, *Crime, Shame and Reintegration* (New York: Cambridge University Press, 1989).

91. Arnold Lubasch, "Chiropractor Given 4-Year Prison Term," *New York Times*, 30 Sept. 1989.

Index

Compositor: Braun-Brumfield, Inc.
Text: 11/14 Electra
Display: Electra
Printer: Braun-Brumfield, Inc.
Binder: Braun-Brumfield, Inc.